Six Countries, Six Reform Models:
The Healthcare Reform
Experience of Israel,
The Netherlands, New Zealand, Singapore,
Switzerland and Taiwan

Healthcare Reforms "Under the Radar Screen"

edited by

Kieke G H Okma

New York University, USA

Luca Crivelli

University of Lugano, Switzerland

with Foreword by **Rudolf Klein**

Six Countries, Six Reform Models: The Healthcare Reform
Experience of Israel, The Netherlands, New Zealand, Singapore, Switzerland and Taiwan

Healthcare Reforms "Under the Radar Screen"

edited by

Kieke G H Okma
New York University, USA

Luca Crivelli
University of Lugano, Switzerland

with Foreword by **Rudolf Klein**

Toni Ashton
University of Auckland, New Zealand

Iva Bolgiani
University of Lugano, Switzerland

Tsung-Mei Cheng
Princeton University, USA

David Chinitz
The Hebrew University of Jerusalem, Israel

Meng-Kin Lim
National University of Singapore, Singapore

Rachel Meislin
Hebrew University-Hadassah, Jerusalem

Hans Maarse
Maastricht University, The Netherlands

Tim Tenbensel
University of Auckland, New Zealand

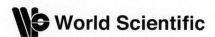
World Scientific

NEW JERSEY · LONDON · SINGAPORE · BEIJING · SHANGHAI · HONG KONG · TAIPEI · CHENNAI

Published by

World Scientific Publishing Co. Pte. Ltd.

5 Toh Tuck Link, Singapore 596224

USA office: 27 Warren Street, Suite 401-402, Hackensack, NJ 07601

UK office: 57 Shelton Street, Covent Garden, London WC2H 9HE

Library of Congress Cataloging-in-Publication Data
Six countries, six reform models--the healthcare reform experience of Israel, the Netherlands,
    New Zealand, Singapore, Switzerland, and Taiwan : healthcare reforms "under the radar screen" /
    edited by Kieke G H Okma ... [et al.].
      p. ; cm.
  Includes bibliographical references and index.
  ISBN-13: 978-9814261586 (hardcover : alk. paper)
  ISBN-10: 9814261580 (hardcover : alk. paper)
  1. Health care reform. I. Okma, Kieke G. H.
  [DNLM: 1. Health Care Reform. 2. Cross-Cultural Comparison. WA 540.1 S625 2009]
  RA394.9.S59 2009
  362.1'0425--dc22

                                                                          2009047318

British Library Cataloguing-in-Publication Data
A catalogue record for this book is available from the British Library.

Typeset by Stallion Press
Email: enquiries@stallionpress.com

Printed in Singapore by B & Jo Enterprise Pte Ltd

Contents

Contents

Foreword

For anyone wondering whether to invest time in reading a new cross-national study of policy making and policy implementation in health care systems, there are three tests. First, does the study provide authoratitive new information? Second, does the new information fit into an existing interpretative framework, so that its findings are not randomly idiosyncratic but add to our existing stock of knowledge and theory? Third, and perhaps the most important, does it have an element of challenge and so provoke reflection about at least some of our assumptions about the dynamics of health care policy making and implementation? In short, the most instructive studies offer a mixture of reassurance and surprise, building on existing theory but also raising new questions.

This study passes all three tests, and offers just the right mix of the predictable and the surprising. The authors of the six national studies are all steeped in the history of the health care systems of their countries. Here there are no examples of intellectual tourism or instant, parachute expertise. So the accounts carry authority, although no doubt the national experience has also shaped the interpretations of the authors (the accounts would be dull indeed if they aspired to that scholarly mirage, total neutrality and objectivity: there is a nice critical edge to most chapters). Further, there is analytic discipline: Explanations of policy change are anchored in the comparative literature, so that common themes run through the chapters. Familiar concepts, like path dependency, provide signposts as we move through unfamiliar territory. And, satisfying my last criterion, the accounts yield interesting puzzles as well as insights about the dynamics of policy making in the health care arena.

The insights and puzzles are, in a sense, independent of any interest in the six specific countries covered by the study. The countries are a remarkably heterogeneous lot. There is no obvious reason why anyone interested in Singapore and Taiwan as examples of health care development in the Asian tiger economies should also be interested in Switzerland and the Netherlands as examples of corporatist style policy making, or in New Zealand and Israel for that matter. And conversely so. The variations between the six are remarkable. In terms of size, they range from under five million to almost 23 million. They include the country with the lowest level of health care expenditure among the rich nations (Singapore, spending 3.3% of GDP) to one of the highest (Switzerland, spending 11.4% of GDP). They range from countries with long national histories to those whose independence is a relatively recent phenomenon. Their constitutions differ, as do their political cultures. Although all can be categorized as rich countries, per capita income in the richest among the six is almost twice that in the least well off.

But it is, of course, precisely these variations which make the one characteristic shared by all six so remarkable. They all have comprehensive health care systems covering the entire population. So the first lesson that can be drawn from this study is that economic determinism is not helpful when explaining the performance of developed health care systems. Singapore with the highest per capita income is also the most frugal health care spender. But conversely, the six also provide a warning against ethnic over-explanation in cultural terms. So while it is tempting to explain Singapore's remarkable performance in terms of "Asian values" — such as the emphasis on family self-reliance — the very different course taken by Taiwan would suggest caution in using this explanatory variable.

On the face of it, of course, there are other similarities. The language of choice and competition has become international in discourse about health policy. It has been invoked in policy debates in all six countries, as elsewhere. But the way it is interpreted, and the degree to which it influences policy outputs, varies from country to country. Ideas can slip across frontiers easily, but institutions are national. If there is any common theme to emerge from the six country studies, it is the extent to which institutions constrain and shape policy making: While they do not determine outcomes, they do set the limits of what is possible. On the one hand, there is the case of policy making in Singapore, a seemingly irresistible and smooth evolutionary process made possible by what is a unique example of single party rule in a democratic polity. On the other hand, there is the case of Switzerland, which remains as an example of a country with multiple veto points (as famously documented by Immergut) where policy making is an obstacle course. But once again the studies provide a warning against facile determinism: The case of New Zealand shows that while institutions do matter to the extent that they permit (or block) rapid policy reverses, they cannot explain the direction of the changes that follow.

So much for ideas and institutions. What about interests? Here the country studies prompt an intriguing puzzle. There is no systematic analysis of the role of interest groups in policy making or implementation, suggesting that they do not play much of a part. Indeed in the case of the Netherlands, the study explicitly notes a decline in the role of interests. Only in New Zealand does the medical profession appears to have been influential, which prompts the question as to why that country is an exception. And there is, of course, a larger question. Interest groups, and the medical profession in particular, have traditionally been the focus of special attention in comparative health care analyses. Why has this changed? Is it because the medical profession and other interest groups have lost ground in the policy arena or because academic fashions have changed or because their influence is to be traced not so much in policy formulation as in policy implementation? And the case of Taiwan, where the medical profession played no role in the creation of the health care system but is now beginning to flex its muscles, prompts a further speculative conclusion: Which is that the role of policy in creating scope for interest groups may be at least as important as the role of interest groups in shaping policy.

Throughout this study the emphasis is as much on how policies work out in practice as on their genesis. It is an approach which pays handsome dividends and provides some notable cautions against accepting conventional assumptions at face value. In particular, the evidence tends to question the assumption that consumer choice (plus provider competition) will necessarily be the engine driving systems to ever greater efficiency. In the Netherlands, individual consumer choice has been statistically almost invisible; in Switzerland consumers stick with their insurers even when other plans offer lower premiums for the same basket of benefits. Loyalty is the norm. Further, competition may actually reduce consumer choice if insurers contract selectively with fewer providers. Does all this matter, however. Another intriguing question looms up: Could the *threat* of consumer exit be enough to produce the desired result ?

This, then, is a study which provides evidence, questions received wisdom and prompts new questions. All of which should encourage the potential reader to plunge in. The experience will be a rewarding one.

Rudolf Klein
Emeritus Professor of Social Policy
Bath University
Visiting Professor
London School of Economics

Acknowledgements

The editors of this book would like to acknowledge three different organizational events that inspired this undertaking. The first are the series of conferences on health care reforms at the Ditchley House in Oxfordshire, England in the early 1990s. Those meetings brought together government officials, politicians, academics and other experts from the United Kingdom, The United States and some other countries. They also provided a platform for well-structured debate on current health reform issues. Some of the participants at the Ditchley House conferences who were inspired to continue the health reform debate in another forum, went on to initiate the so-called Four Country Conferences and formed a Steering Committee: Ted Marmor from the U.S. Michael Decter and Carolyn Tuohy from Canada, Martin Pfaff from Germany and Kieke Okma from The Netherlands. Those meetings, sponsored by the governments and other agencies of each of the four countries (and in one case, the Australian government as well), took place between 1995 and 2005. The Four Country Conferences focused their debate issues on health politics in the United States, Canada, Germany and The Netherlands (in a later stage, the editors decided to add the United Kingdom as an important source of policy inspiration). A selected number of conference papers became the base for a book to be published by Yale University Press (at the time of this writing, the book manuscript is with the publisher's for printing). This book discusses both methodological issues of cross-national comparison as well as substantive policy areas, including hospital care, primary care, pharmaceutical policies and long-term care for the elderly. The idea for this comparative book is to include a limited number of countries (small countries bordering large ones) with similar structural features of their health politics, facing similar policy problems and seeking solutions in a similar range of options within their own country-specific health policy arena.

The third venue that inspired the editors of this book was a meeting of a health policy group of the German Bertelsmann Foundation held in Helsinki in 2006. Here, the two editors of this volume (representing smaller countries themselves) met and agreed to collaborate on research that would focus on smaller countries' health reform experiences. Some other participants at that meeting joined in the project, too. It first resulted in an article about the health reform experiences of Chile, Israel, Singapore, Switzerland, Taiwan and The Netherlands (accepted by the *Journal of Comparative Policy Analysis*). Next, this collaborative effort expanded to include New Zealand as well. The editors thus acknowledge the Ditchley House Foundation, the series of Four Country Conferences and the Bertelsmann Foundation as their inspirational sources.

Next, the editors would like to express their gratitude to Meryl Schwartz for her extensive editorial support. Meryl has worked hard to transform raw drafts into eloquent language and also helped to collect and present the data in the statistical Appendix to this book. We also like to thank Sook-Cheng Lim of World Scientific Publishers in Singapore who patiently accepted delays and remained very supportive of the project.

Finally, the editors acknowledge that without the enthusiastic support and contributions by their co-authors they would not have been able to cook this book, so to say, within the surprisingly short period of time of less than two years.

About the Authors

Kieke Okma received her PhD from the University Utrecht in 1997. She has worked with a variety of government agencies in The Netherlands and abroad for over 25 years. Since 2004, she has lived in New York and works as an international health consultant and academic. She is Associate Professor (adjunct) at the Wagner School of Public Services, New York University and Visiting Professor at the Catholic University, Leuven. She is on the editorial boards of *Health Policy*, the *Journal of Health Politics, Policy and Law* and the *Journal of Health Services, Research and Policy*. Kieke Okma has lectured widely and published on a broad range of health policy issues, including health politics, and international comparison. Recent publications include "Recent Changes in Dutch Health Insurance: Individual Mandate or Social Health Insurance?" (Paper), Annual Meeting, National Academy of Social Insurance, 2008; "Comparative Perspectives on National Values, Institutions and Health Policies" (with Theodore R. Marmor and Stephen R. Latham) in *Sociology of Health and Illness*, C. Wendt, ed. 2006; "Comparative Perspectives and Policy Learning in the World of Health Care" (with T.R. Marmor and R. Freeman); "Health Care Systems in Transition of the World Health Organization" (with T.R Marmor, book review essay); "The Method of Open Co-ordination: Open Procedures or Closed Circuit?" *European Journal of Social Security*, 2002; "What is the Best Public-Private Model for Canadian Health Care?" (Paper), Montreal: Institute for Research on Public Policy, 2002.

Luca Crivelli received his PhD in Economics from the University of Zurich and is currently Professor of Economics at the University of Applied Sciences of Southern Switzerland and Adjunct Professor at the University of Lugano. Since 1999, he has been director of Net-MEGS, a masters program in health economics and management organized by the University of

Lugano, and since 2005, he has been a member of the extended management board of the Swiss School of Public Health. In 2004, he joined the international health policy and reform network sponsored by the Bertelsmann Foundation as an expert and policy analyst for Switzerland. From 2004 to 2007, he was part of the advisory committee of the Swiss conference of cantonal health ministers covering the ongoing reforms of Swiss health insurance. Crivelli has published peer-reviewed articles on cross-border care (*Swiss Journal of Economics and Statistics*), regulation of pharmaceutical markets (*Journal of Regulatory Economics*), federalism and health expenditure (*Health Economics*), efficiency of health care institutions (*International Journal of Health Care Finance and Economics*) and reforms of health insurance in Switzerland (*Revue française des affaires sociales*).

Toni Ashton (PhD) is an Associate Professor in Health Economics and Director of the Centre for Health Services Research and Policy in the School of Population Health, University of Auckland, New Zealand. Her primary field of research and publication is in the analysis of the organization and funding of health systems with a special focus on health care reform. Having worked in the field for over 20 years, she has been a member of a number of government working parties covering various aspects of health policy, and is on the editorial board of four academic journals. She has also consulted extensively for international agencies such as WHO and OECD, and nationally for government agencies, health professional bodies, and non-government organizations.

Iva Bolgiani received her PhD in Economic and Social Sciences from the University of Geneva and now works as a scientific consultant at the Sezione sanitaria in the Canton of Ticino, with a special focus on quality improvement programs for hospitals and contracting with the public cantonal hospitals. She is a member of the teaching staff at the Universities of Geneva, Lausanne and Lugano. She has served as external expert of the national commission on health prevention and communication and she is a member of several inter-cantonal commissions working on health policy issues at the national level. She has published several articles in both

Swiss and international journals, and one book. She also collaborates with the HPM program of the Bertelsmann Foundation.

David Chinitz received his BA with the Bennett Prize in Political Science from Columbia College in 1973, and his PhD in Public Policy Analysis from the University of Pennsylvania in 1981. After moving to Israel in 1981, he has held positions as Head of the Division of Social Sciences in the Israeli Ministry of Science; Senior Researcher at the JDC/Brookdale Institute in Jerusalem; and Senior Lecturer in the Department of Health Policy and Management of the Hebrew University-Hadassah School of Public Health. He has been a visiting scholar at the Schools of Public Health of Columbia University and the University of California, Berkeley, as well as the Wagner School of Public Service, New York University. He is immediate past Scientific Chair of the European Health Management Association and a member of the Management Board of the International Society for Priorities in Health Care, and serves on the editorial board of a number of health and public health journals and as a consultant to the World Health Organization. David Chinitz has edited several books and authored numerous articles and chapters on comparative health systems, health policy and regulation, and quality assurance.

Rudolf Klein, CBE, was born in Prague. After graduating from Oxford, he spent the first half of his career as a journalist with the *London Evening Standard* and *The Observer*. From 1978 to 1998 he was Professor of Social Policy at Bath University and is currently Visiting Professor at the London School of Economics and the London School of Hygiene. He is a Senior Fellow of the British Academy, a Fellow of the Academy of Medical Sciences, and a Foreign Associate of the Institute of Medicine. Apart from *The New Politics of the NHS* (5th edition, 2006), he has written several books about accountability, consumer representation and rationing, as well as many articles about public policy in academic and other journals.

Meng K Lim is Associate Professor of Health Policy and Management at the Yong Loo Lin School of Medicine, National University of

Singapore. He is also the Academic Director of the Master of Business Administration (Healthcare Management) Program at the NUS Business School and Director of Public Health of the Association of Pacific Rim Universities World Institute (http://www.apru.org/awi). A physician by training, Dr. Lim was Chief of the Singapore Armed Forces Medical Corps (1986–1995); Founding Director of the Defense Medical Research Institute (1994–1997), and Chief Executive Officer of the Health Corporation of Singapore (1997–1999). He has served on several hospital boards and numerous expert commissions. Dr. Lim has published over 80 scientific articles in international, peer-reviewed journals — including *New England Journal of Medicine*, *Health Affairs*, *Health Policy*, *Medical Care*, *Quality and Safety in Health Care*, *Journal of Health Policy, Politics and Law*, *British Medical Journal*, and *British Journal of Public Health Medicine*. He is Editorial Board Member of *Health Services Research*, *Health Research Policy and Systems*, and *Asian Journal of Health and Information Sciences*. He is also Scientific Committee Member of the International Academy of Aviation and Space Medicine. Internationally, Dr. Lim has represented Singapore on the WHO Western Pacific Advisory Committee on Health Research and the International Network on Healthcare Reform. He has also consulted extensively for the World Bank, WHO, Asian Development Bank, as well as the Ministries of Health of Singapore, China, Vietnam, Thailand, Indonesia, Malaysia, Brunei, Hong Kong, Iran, Lebanon, Egypt, West Bank, Gaza, Kuwait, and Bulgaria. Among his awards are the Republic of Singapore's Public Service Star and the Public Administration (Silver) Medal. In 2004, he received the NUS Special Commendation Award for Teaching Excellence.

Hans Maarse is an expert in health policy and administration. After his receiving his PhD in political science, he worked for 10 years at the Faculty of Public Administration at Twente University. Since 1986, he has been a professor in the Faculty of Health Sciences at the University of Maastricht. He has consulted frequently for the WHO and the World Bank. His current fields of interest are the impact of the EU on health policy-making, comparative health systems analysis, and market reforms in healthcare systems (in particular, The Netherlands). He has recently published on these topics in the *Journal of Health Politics, Policy and Law, Health Care Analysis, Health Policy, the European Journal of Health Economics, EuroHealth, Journal of Medicine and Philosophy, BMC Health Services Research, Intereconomics* and in several books on healthcare policymaking. He is also a member or chairman of the supervisory boards of several healthcare provider organizations in The Netherlands.

Rachel Meislin is a recent graduate of the University of Pennsylvania with a BA in Health and Societies, and has interned as a research associate at the Department of Health Policy and Management, School of Public Health, Hebrew University-Hadassah, Jerusalem. She is currently pursuing a career in medicine.

Tsung-Mei Cheng is an expert on comparative health systems with an emphasis on Asian countries. Cheng writes and lectures internationally on topics ranging from single payer systems, health systems change, health care quality, financing, pay for performance focusing on East Asian health systems, to the impact of the WTO and GATS on national health policy. She is the co-founder of the Princeton Conference, an annual national conference on health policy that brings together the U.S. Congress, government, and the research community on issues affecting health care and health policy in the United States. Cheng is an adviser to the China Health Economics Institute, the official government think tank for health policy under China's Ministry of Health charged with, among other things, conducting policy-oriented research on national health care development strategy and health care system reform and provide policy recommendations to policy makers. She is also an advisor to NICE International, an agency of the National Institute for Health and Clinical Excellence that advises the National Health Service (NHS) of the United Kingdom on NHS coverage decisions and clinical and public health guidelines, as well as a member of the International Advisory Group of Academy Health, the US-based professional association of health services researchers, and a board member of the America-China Medical Association. Cheng was an adviser in 2003 to the Strategic Review Board of the Science and Technology Advisory Group (STAG), a body charged with advising the Office of the Premier of Taiwan, on the development of science and technology. Currently she is working on cross-national comparisons of health systems in East Asia focusing on health reforms in China and Taiwan. Cheng is the host, writer, and executive editor of the "International Forum," a Princeton University television program on international affairs focusing on global political, economic, security issues as well as issues concerning global health.

Tim Tenbensel is a senior lecturer in health policy at the School of Population Health, University of Auckland, New Zealand. He is assistant editor of Social Science and Medicine, and a member of the Advisory Board for the *Policy & Politics Journal*. Recent publications include "How Do Governments Steer Health Policy? A Comparison of Canadian and New Zealand Approaches to Cost-Control and Primary Health Care Reform," *Journal of Comparative Policy Analysis* **10**, no. 4 (forthcoming). "Public Health Sciences and Policy in High Income Countries" (with Peter Davis) In *Oxford Textbook of Public Health*, eds. Roger Detels, Robert Beaglehole, Mary-Ann Lansang, and Martin Guilford. Oxford: Oxford University Press (forthcoming). "Where There's a Will, Is There A Way?" (with J. Cumming, T. Ashton, and P. Barnett), *Social Science and Medicine* **67**, no. 7: 1143–1152, 2008. "Decentralizing Resource Allocation: Early Experiences with District Health Boards in New Zealand" (with T. Ashton, J. Cumming, and P. Barnett) *Journal of Health Services Research and Policy* **13**, no. 2: 109–115, 2008. "Policy Knowledge for Policy Work." In *The Work of Policy: An International Survey*, H. K. Colebatch, ed. Lanham: Lexington Books, 2006. "Interest Groups." In *New Zealand Government and Politics*, Raymond Miller, ed. 4th edition. Auckland: Oxford University Press: 525–535, 2006. "Multiple Modes of Governance: Disentangling the Alternatives to Hierarchies and Markets," *Public Management Review* **7**, no. 2: 267–288, 2005, 2004. "Does More Evidence Lead to Better Policy? The Implications of Explicit Priority-Setting in New Zealand's Health Policy for Evidence-Based Policy," *Policy Studies* **25**, no. 3: 189–207, 2004.

Introduction

Kieke G. H. Okma and Luca Crivelli

This book presents a diagnosis of the health reform experiences of six small and midsize industrial democracies — Israel, The Netherlands, New Zealand, Singapore, Switzerland, and Taiwan — during the last two decades of the 20th century.[1] The countries span the globe, hailing from Asia, the Middle East, and Europe. The study seeks to contribute to cross-national policy learning by structured multicountry research. It looks at the health reform experiences of six quite different health care systems. In that sense, it represents a "most different system design" (Marmor, 1988), under a common analytical framework.

At first glance, the countries selected for this comparative study do not have much in common. They are located on different continents and vary greatly in size, population, ethnicity, and historical background (see the tables in the Appendix for statistical data on size, populations, income levels, economic growth, and health expenditure). The countries differ in dominant cultural orientations and economic circumstances, with very different traditions and styles of socioeconomic and fiscal policy-making.

[1] This study has its roots in an article for the *Journal of Comparative Policy Analysis* that the authors wrote in 2008. That contribution became the base for this more extended study. During the process of transforming an article into the book format, we added New Zealand as an interesting laboratory for change in health governance. Unfortunately, due to unforeseen events, we had to drop Chile as a full chapter in this volume. However, given the striking experiences in Chile — in particular, the sweeping policy shifts after the military takeover in 1973, and again after the return to democracy in 1990 — we refer to that country in referencing "exclusionary policy-making." We would like to express our gratitude to Eliana Labra for her collaboration.

However, they also have some important features in common. They all are small-to-midsize industrialized democracies with open economies.[2] They share the general policy goal of providing universal access to good quality health care, and all six have sought to broaden insurance coverage while restraining public expenditure. Over time, they have faced similar fiscal strains (with the notable exception of Singapore), growing (and changing) demand for medical services, and shifting perceptions of the role of the state in society. Moreover, all have discussed a similar range of reform options, and all have enlarged access to health care services by expanding (public and private) health insurance.

Another common feature of the group is that — illustrating the need to make a careful distinction between policy as *intentions* or *plans* and policy as *implemented* change (Palmer and Short, 1989) — they actually undertook major reforms in the last two decades, rather than just discussing policy intentions. Public discontent with existing arrangements, combined with the availability of policy options and political willingness to act, created "windows of opportunity" (Kingdon, 1984) for such change. Finally, and perhaps most importantly, the cases selected fall somewhat "under the radar screen": they are not usually included in international comparative studies

---

[2] One question we have not addressed extensively in this book is: What counts as a "small" or "medium"-size country? Most international comparative studies take one or more of the world's largest industrialized countries as the main comparator: the United States, the United Kingdom, Canada, Germany, France, and sometimes other OECD member states. We use the term "small and medium-sized" to indicate countries that clearly do not belong to that group. In the introduction to his grand oeuvre, *Rich Democracies*, Harold Wilensky (2002) discusses the size issue. He argues that rather than the actual size in terms of the population or geographic area, it is the complexity of administration that matters. The countries studied in this book all have long traditions of public health care funding and contracting, under a variety of (complex) administrative arrangements. However, there is one other common feature of policy-making in small countries that is worth noting: the small size of the market and policy arena creates strong barriers to exit. First, there is much personal overlap in the health care field (such as board membership of hospitals or health insurance combined with political functions or expert advisorships); in the health policy arena, the major players know each other personally. Moreover, health care is mostly "local." The findings of this study also confirm that most people do not want to travel long distances to obtain medical care, nor can they move to another town or region easily. This also limits the "consumer exit."

(even while there has been a recent surge of interest in the experiences of Switzerland and Holland — see Naik, 2007; Harris, 2007; Herzlinger and Parsa-Parsi, 2004; Reinhardt 2004; Leu *et al.*, 2009).

This book addresses the following questions: Why have the six countries of this study, facing similar pressures to reform their health care systems and with similar options for government action, chosen very different pathways to restructure their health care? What caused a "window of opportunity" (Kingdon, 1984) for change in each case? What did they do? What was the position of the major stakeholders? And what happened after the implementation of those reforms? How did patients, health insurers, and health care providers choose and change their "voice" and "exit" strategies (Hirschman, 1970)?

This introductory chapter addresses some of the methodological issues of international comparison, especially the issue of categorizing countries, health systems, and health policies. It next summarizes the main findings of this study.

The following chapters analyze the health care reform experiences of Isráel, The Netherlands, New Zealand, Singapore, Switzerland, and Taiwan during the last two decades of the 20th century and the beginning of the 21st century. Those chapters provide a brief overview of the historical developments of the health care systems, and the current arrangements for funding, contracting, payment, ownership, and adminis-tration (or "governance") of health care. They address the origins of the health care reforms, the external and internal pressures for change, the discussion of policy options, the processes of implementation, and the often-neglected but almost universal "post-reform adjustments."

The final chapter of the book discusses both the empirical findings and general conclusions about comparative methodology. The Appendix pro-vides statistical data on each country's size, population, economic growth, income levels, and health care spending. It also contains an overview of the dominant cultural orientations and modes of governance in health care.

The study is a truly international collaboration. The authors have all lived and worked in one or more of these countries, combining a variety of academic and administrative backgrounds with personal experiences.

They brought together a unique degree of in-depth knowledge that allowed for more detailed findings than studies solely based on the Organization for Economic Cooperation and Development's (OECD) aggregate data, or data from similar international sources. This has greatly improved our understanding of similarities and differences between the national experiences.

The conclusions of this book confirm the need to collaborate across countries and disciplines. No individual researcher can do a systematic study of change and nonchange in, say, more than three or four countries at this depth of understanding and detail. Second, the study confirms the need to pay more attention to small and medium-size countries. Most of the comparative research in the field focuses on big countries, with the United Sates, Canada, the United Kingdom, and sometimes France, Germany, Japan, and Australia among the usual suspects. There is far less research on the experiences of small and midsize countries, while, in fact, the vast majority of the world's nations fall into this category. To fill this gap, many more studies are needed. This research aims to take a step in that direction.

Analytical Frameworks

Harold Lasswell's famous book (1936), *Politics*, summarizes the essentials of public policy: Who gets what, when, how? In health politics, those essential questions translate into a wide range of public activities, including the direct provision of some public health services, research funding, medical education, regulating health professionals, protecting patients and the general public, and safeguarding access to health care services by spreading the costs of medical care across populations to protect family income against insurmountable costs of illness. The mechanisms for spreading the costs (or "pooling risks") of health care across large populations require public action to define the populations that have access to certain schemes, to define the entitlements under public coverage, to determine the level of contributions and other financial conditions, and to set rules for administration and monitoring the outcomes of the system. Private markets can pool risks, too, but on a limited scale. In the private market, the insured face premiums that reflect their actuarial risk (expected future costs): the higher the risk, the higher the premium. Persons with certain medical conditions (such as a chronic illness or disability) may be denied coverage altogether. Community-rating in private insurance is based on segmentation of insured into more or less homogenous groups. In contrast, public health insurance offers coverage to populations regardless of their medical conditions, charges contributions based on their ability to pay, and aims to provide access to medical treatment without undue barriers to all who need care. Community-rating under social health insurance ignores the actuarial risk of the individual, but instead spreads payment across the wider populations via general taxation or income-related contributions for mandated social insurance.

Most industrialized countries share basic underlying principles and goals — sometimes solely rhetorical — in health policy: universal (or near-universal) access to health services and health insurance, solidarity (understood as fairness) in sharing the financial burden of medical treatment, and good quality of services (OECD, 1992).[3]

---

[3] In the context of health insurance, the term "solidarity" — often taken as "equity" — translates into quite divergent arrangements. It generally refers to the sharing of the financial burden of health insurance. In a narrow (most-commonly-used and least-questioned) sense, "equity" means that everybody faces the same burden, and has access to medical services when he or she needs them. The measure for "the same burden" usually is taken as the same share of family income; thus, proportional tax is fully equal, while community-rated flat premiums are regressive, with higher income groups paying a lower share of their incomes than people with lower incomes. Another interpretation of "equity," however, takes equity as a commonsense notion of fairness, namely the absence of insurmountable financial barriers to health care. For example, the early European sick funds charged the same contributions to all their members and offered equal medical services to all. Likewise, until recently, all members of a particular sick fund in Germany paid the same contribution rates (but the rates differed from fund to fund). The community-rating served as an equalization mechanism between the members, not between the funds. In contrast (until 2006), members of sick funds in The Netherlands all paid the same income-dependent contribution, plus a modest flat-rate premium per person. The British NHS gets most of its funding from general taxation; the degree of equity thus depends on the redistributive working of the tax system. These are three examples of funding mechanisms that general populations perceive as fair or equitable, even while the distributional effects are often not.

With a growing public share in health care funding, increasing efficiency and cost control has become one of the overriding concerns of governments. Most nations regard patient satisfaction, patient choice, and professional autonomy of physicians as important goals, too.[4]

Nonetheless, there is wide variety in the funding and contracting mechanisms of health care. For example, in Canada, Australia, Italy, New Zealand, the United Kingdom, Italy, Spain, and the Scandinavian countries, the major share of health care funding comes out of general taxation. In Austria, Belgium, Germany, France, Luxembourg, and The Netherlands, social (and, to a lesser degree, private) health insurance systems are the main source. In all countries, patients pay for some health care out of their own pockets or face copayments for other services. In most cases, however, governments have mitigated the effects of user fees by exempting certain groups or setting annual limits on the amount that families must pay (rather than, as is common in private health insurance, setting limits on how much reimbursement families can receive each year).

The variation in funding and contracting models in health care can be traced to country-specific historical developments. Two particular events in Europe played a crucial role. The first was the 1883 introduction of social health insurance for industrial workers and their dependents in Germany by Chancellor Bismarck; the legislation required that all industrial workers and their families become members of a sick

---

[4] The notion of "consumer choice" in health care has taken on different meanings. For most patients and in most countries, "choice" refers to their ability to see a physician or other health care provider of their choice. In modern day health policy-making, the term commonly refers to the possibility of signing up with a health insurance or health plan of one's choice. Paradoxically, the increased choice of plan sometimes reduces the choice of provider: when insurers can selectively contract, their insured may find that their particular plan has not contracted their regular or preferred provider — say, their long-standing family physician or dentist.

fund.[5] The effect was that sick funds had more stable revenue streams and could create wider risk pools. In the 20th century, sick funds became core actors in the public policy arena, sharing the responsibility for social policy-making, but also facing more and more government regulation.

The second major innovation in the funding of health care in the 20th century was the establishment of Britain's National Health Service (NHS) in 1948 (Klein, 2005; Timmins, 1995).[6] The NHS extended the German

---

[5] That step raised great interest in many, if not all, industrialized countries across the globe. Several countries in Europe — and some in Latin America and Asia as well — followed the German example of state-sponsored (but not state-administered), mandatory social insurance to protect the families of industrial workers against the financial risks of illness, disability, unemployment, and old age. The unique feature of the Bismarckian scheme of 1883 was that it built on the existing institutions of the 19th century mutual societies, or sick funds, which, in turn, could already be traced back to the Middle Ages (De Swaan, 1988; Daschel, 2008). Bismarck did not replace those sick funds, but made membership mandatory for certain categories of workers. The sick funds (commonly but somewhat mistakenly labeled as "sickness funds"; the literal translation of the original, German term "*Krankenkassen*" means "fund of — and for — the sick") remained legally independent, risk-bearing insurers for members and their families. Labor unions' representatives, workers, and employers all sat on the sick funds' boards. Each fund set its own premium (usually shared between worker and employer on a 50–50 basis). The funds offered modest amounts of income replacement in case of illness, disability, unemployment, or old age of the breadwinner. They also provided health services for their members, as they employed physicians and set up clinics.

[6] In 1943, an expert committee headed by Beveridge presented a model for the entire system of social security after the war. It advocated a health system that would extend access to health care to the entire population by paying services out of general taxation and nationalizing health facilities. The war itself contributed to the creation of a "window of opportunity" (Kingdon, 1984): for the first time in history, members of different social classes met in times of duress; they had shared the underground shelters during air raids, for example, and were therefore ready to acknowledge that every person needed health care, regardless of income or background. The Beveridge report argued that the additional investments in hospitals and other services would only be temporary. The underlying assumption was that such investments would ultimately reduce public health expenditure, as it would help wounded war veterans and disabled workers return to the labor force as soon as possible. The nationalization of hospitals gave the government the say (and financial responsibility) on investing in expanding the capacity of hospital care. In the postwar decades, there was some concern about costs, but the NHS had become very popular. It did deliver on its promise of universal health care, albeit in a frugal way. And, once in place, it had created its own constituencies which helped to shape the almost "untouchable" position of the NHS for decades (Pierson, 1999).

insurance model by providing coverage to the entire population, paid out of general taxation. While nationalizing hospitals, the NHS retained the status of family physicians as independent practitioners.[7]

In the first half of the 20th century, several countries in Western Europe followed the German example and implemented one or more income protection schemes for certain groups in society (for example, disability and unemployment benefits for industrial workers). It was only after World War II, however, that they developed a full range of modern welfare state arrangements, including old age pensions, disability and unemployment benefits, health insurance, sickness pay, and child support. In the first two decades after World War II, there was strong popular support for this expansion of state-sponsored schemes. Some countries followed the German example of employment-based schemes, while others preferred the population-wide NHS model. The spread of the two models was not restricted to Europe. Nations across the world sought to implement similar arrangements to protect the incomes of their populations (or population groups) against the financial risks of illness, disability, and old age. By the end of the 20th century, most, if not all, countries' health care funding had become hybridized, incorporating elements of both the German and the UK model by combining employment-based arrangements for certain categories of workers with population-wide and tax-based universal schemes. This hybridization has important consequences for efforts to place countries in categories (see below).

The 1970s saw a rather sudden turnabout from expansion and popular support for the welfare state arrangements to reassessment and retrenchment. A confluence of economic, demographic, and ideological factors contributed to reshaping the popular notion of the welfare state from a *solution* for social problems to a *cause* of economic stagnation and an economic burden (Wilensky, 2002; Marmor, Mashaw, and Harvey, 1990; Timmins, 1995). Economic stagnation in conjunction with persistent and

---

[7] Almost ten years before the creation of the NHS in 1948, hospital care in New Zealand had already become a universal entitlement for the entire population, paid out of general taxation.

high levels of unemployment following the oil crises of the 1970s meant that state incomes stagnated or declined while public spending continued to grow. Moreover, as the end of the postwar baby boom became apparent, demographers realized that they had to revise their earlier demographic projections downward (and future pension outlays upward).

Adding to these economic and demographic pressures, there had been a marked ideological change regarding the role of the state. On both the left and the right of the political spectrum, critics agreed that state powers had become too wide, too dominant, and too intrusive in the lives of individuals. Existing welfare arrangements were challenged by growing discontent over fiscal burdens, disappointing results of public programs, rising consumerism, and patient advocacy groups claiming a stronger say in the allocation and organization of health care. These factors also fueled an extensive search by governments for alternative governance models that could reduce the dominant role of the state, decentralize decision-making, and provide more room for individual choice and entrepreneurial ideas (Ranade, 1998; Cutler, 2002). Some countries took hesitant steps to introduce market competition in health care, reducing state control over the funding and planning of health care services (such as determining hospital capacity, or the numbers of local general practitioners). They also sought to broaden the choice of provider and health plan for patients and the insured. Other countries turned to traditional tools for controlling public expenditure by setting strict budgets, reducing the scope of public insurance, and increasing direct patient payments.

The above internal and external pressures for change also encouraged national governments to look elsewhere for solutions and new ideas: "No one wants to be caught wearing yesterday's ideas," Rudolf Klein (1995) once observed. This search for new ideas fueled a rapid proliferation of cross-national studies in the field of health policy in the 1980s and 1990s. The majority of those comparative studies, however, consist of collections of *descriptive* case studies based on aggregate national statistics. They often lack a common vocabulary or focus, and suffer from poorly defined terms (Marmor and Okma, 2003). For example, terms like "health reform," "managed competition" or "consumer-driven health care" are regularly used, but rarely defined in any operational way. Many comparative studies aim to analyze processes of health reform across the globe, but few pay attention to what it is, conceptually, they seek to explain.[8]

Another common mistake is the assumption that policy as stated in formal government documents or law is the same as policy actually implemented. As we will demonstrate, for a variety of reasons the ultimate outcome of reform often differs greatly from original policy intentions and statements. Faced with public discontent over (intended or unintended) results, governments often feel pressured to adjust their policies.

In this contribution, we take "health reform" as major shifts in both decision-making powers over the allocation of resources, and financial risks in the funding, contracting, ownership, and administration (or governance) of health care. Such shifts include the abolition (or reinstatement) of selective contracting with providers, changes in the authority over capital investments, and expansion or contraction of public health insurance entitlements. They can also include (new) restrictions on medical decision-making imposed by practice guidelines and other rules. Further, decision-making power and financial risks can shift from the national level to regional and local governments (or in the other direction), or from government control to health insurers, individual patients, and the insured.

The main focus of this study is on changes in health insurance, medical care provided in hospitals, and individual medical practices, including prescription drugs and medical aids. However, the borderline between medical care and related social services (such as long-term care for the elderly or disabled) is not always clear, and countries have different views on what constitutes "health care." Another limitation of

---

[8] "Governance," another example of a conceptually fuzzy term, is a rising star in today's terminology. Basically, it refers to the administration of health insurance and health care. Interestingly, it has traveled from the government to the corporate sector and back to the public sector (Okma, 2002: footnotes 14 and 18). During this migration, it also shed its neutral meaning and took on a normative connotation under the label "good governance" and, more recently, "stewardship." In this contribution, we take "governance" in a neutral sense: administration (both public and private) of health services and health insurance.

this study is its main focuses: health policies aimed at protecting family incomes against financial risks of illness, and policies to improve the organization of health care services. Because of these focuses, it pays less attention to policies that predominantly or exclusively aim to improve the health of the population (such as by improving road safety, food quality, consumer protection, or changes in lifestyle).

The study combines analytical categories from economic theory with concepts from political science. The economic terms describe the basic constituent elements of health care systems: the funding, contracting, and provision of health services. The terms borrowed from political science serve to analyze the "workings" of the health care system and the behavior of the main actors: governments, patients, the insured, health insurers, and providers of health care services. Klein and Marmor (2006) argue that the major models of political science fall under three broad headings: ideas, interests, and institutions. Those terms refer to underlying social values (or "dominant cultural orientations"), organized stakeholders in society, and political institutions that shape social policy in all countries.

The selection and combination of the aforementioned analytical frameworks is, by its very nature, somewhat eclectic. There is no common vocabulary across the different disciplines, and there is no generally accepted hierarchy of public policy theories (Okma, 1997a). Nonetheless, the wider selection of theoretical frameworks for this study (discussed below) has proven useful for examining the six countries' health reform experiences because it has allowed a systematic comparison of some of the core features of their health care systems as well as the causes and consequences of varied policy change.

According to reports of the OECD, it is possible to describe any given health care system in terms of a country-specific mix of public and private funding, contracting, and modes of providing medical services (OECD, 1992, 1994). In general, there are five main sources of funding and three dominant contracting models. The major funding sources are general taxation (general revenues, earmarked taxes, and tax expenditure), public and private insurance, direct patient payments (copayments, coinsurance, deductibles, and uninsured services), and voluntary contributions. For some developing countries, external aid can be a major source as well.

There are three basic contracting models in health care. The first is the "integrated model," with funding and ownership of services under the same (public or private) responsibility. The best-known example of this model is the original British National Health Service (NHS) of 1948. The NHS provided tax-funded health care for all, largely paid out of general taxation. A modern-day example of an integrated private model is the health maintenance organization (HMO) in the United States (at least, the original form of the Kaiser Permanente HMO).[9] In fact, that model closely resembles the 19th century German sick funds that owned clinics and employed physicians to provide health services to their members. The second model is the "contracting model," where governments or other third party payers (mostly the administrative agencies of social health insurance and, in some cases, private health insurers) negotiate long-term contracts with health care providers. The third funding model (or, rather, payment model), common in private insurance, is that of reimbursement, where the patient first pays his provider and then seeks reimbursement from his insurance agency.

On the provision side, the ownership and management of health services can be public, private (both for-profit and not-for-profit), or — in most countries — a mix of the two. Moreover, there are country-specific mixes of formal and informal care, traditional and modern medicine, and medical and related social services. In this contribution, the emphasis is on medical care but, as we stated earlier, borderlines with other services are

---

[9] It is important to note that the term "health maintenance organization," or HMO, includes a variety of organizational models (Hacker and Marmor, 2007). In the 1970s, HMOs were heralded as organizations that would help contain health expenditure in the US by selectively and critically contracting health services on behalf of their insured. Over time, HMOs faced increased dissatisfaction of insured and physicians over such restrictions (e.g. the gag rules that prohibited physicians from discussing the terms of their contracts with others, or the limited lengths of stays allowed for women after childbirth). More and more states passed law to restrain the restrainers, and many HMOs changed strategy by shifting risks to groups of providers based on capitated payments for a certain group of patients.

not always clear, and national health policies reflect divergent cultural views about such borderlines.

The combination of those three core elements — funding, contracting (including the payment modes), and ownership — largely determines the allocation of financial risks and decision-making power over the main players in health care. For example, the risk-rated premiums of private insurance expose low-income families to higher costs than social insurance (particularly because level of income often correlates with health status: the lower the income, the poorer the health of population groups). Moreover, private insurance may require families to pay more out of pocket by restricting reimbursement, or excluding coverage of some conditions altogether. Social insurance, with income-related premiums and without exclusions, reduces such financial risks for families. As another example, tax funding and government ownership make for strong government influence, whereas private funding (insurance and direct patient payments) combined with legally independent providers shifts the decision-making power to insurers and providers of health care (as in Switzerland or The Netherlands). This is so even while governments can — and often do — impose rules to protect patients or safeguard the quality of and access to health care (for example, by deciding whether to include dental care for adults, contraceptive care, mental health care, or home care in the entitlements of social health insurance).

The above economic terms help to characterize certain features of health care systems and policy-making. They do not explain the *causes* or *effects* of policy change (but can point to the fact that certain features will allow for change more rapidly and more easily than others). In trying to understand why countries have embarked on particular reform paths, we have to look not only at the external and internal pressures for change, but also at the structural features of social policy-making and particular events in time that enable politicians and other policy entrepreneurs to change the system.

OECD countries have developed a variety of administrative or governance models in health care and health insurance. Douglas and Wildavsky (1982) have identified three dominant cultural orientations in welfare states: hierarchical collectivism, competitive individualism, and sectarianism.[10] The first refers to the social-democratic states of northwestern Europe that have based their fiscal and social policy on principles of solidarity and equality. They have collectivist traditions, with strong bureaucratic traditions to implement policy. In some countries, particularly Germany and The Netherlands, those bureaucracies engage in semipermanent "neocorporatist" consultations with organized stakeholders (though this practice has declined in the last two decades in The Netherlands; see the chapter in this volume). The United States, in contrast, is generally seen as being more of a liberal welfare state, with a strong emphasis on competition, individual rights and responsibilities, weak collectivism, and an outspoken streak of sectarianism. Market competition and individual liberty are guiding principles in much of its social policy. In The Netherlands, the neocorporatist tradition was also influenced by religious sectarianism, as many of the associations that played a major role in Dutch politics had religious backgrounds (Lijphart, 1968).

Corresponding with — and adding to — the above three models, which refer to the way government and interest groups in society interact, are the labels (semi-) "pluralist," (semi-) "corporatist," and "exclusionary," which refer to modes of policy-making (Labra, 2007). Douglas and Wildavsky's individualistic orientation corresponds with notions of pluralism, and their hierarchical collectivist orientation with corporatist

[10] Another categorization of social policy takes the underlying welfare principles as starting points: income protection, behaviorist, residualist, and populist redistributive (Marmor, Mashaw, and Harvey, 1990). Income protection is the basic principle of social insurance: it mandates certain groups (or the entire population) to contribute according to their ability to pay, and provides all participants with entitlements according to their needs. Behaviorist policies seek to change the behavior of recipients. For example, it encourages welfare recipients to actively seek employment. The basic idea behind residualist principles is that individuals and families are responsible for their own economic support and the state will step in only as a last resort; for example, low levels (or short duration) of unemployment or disability benefits as a condition for receiving income support. The redistributive policies aim to spread resources amongst populations; for example, education policies may aim to raise the general level of education so that everybody can benefit. These underlying principles (similar to the "dominant cultural orientations") translate into certain styles of policy-making and governance in health care.

styles. The exclusionary mode, however, indicates the power of a strong central government (in the extreme form, a military dictatorship like that of Pinochet in Chile from 1973 to 1990) to exclude certain groups from decision-making over social policy. We will come across examples of all of these policy styles in this book.

It would be an error, however, to assume that such orientations provide an entirely accurate representation of a particular country. Models do not cover countries on a one-to-one basis. Different styles of governance can exist simultaneously, and over time there may be shifts from one style to another (see also the Appendix\of this volume). For example, in the 1980s and 1990s, Dutch health policies shifted from a solidarity-based model toward a hybridized model with elements of market competition, stronger behaviorist principles, and a more residualist role of the state in unemployment and disability policies (see footnote 9 for an explanation of those terms). Still, strong popular support for universal access to health care (and for solidarity in the distribution of the financial burdens) has restrained the efforts of governments to shift to privatized health care. Taiwan, as we will demonstrate, went in the opposite direction by transforming its existing public health insurance schemes into a population-wide national insurance. The Swiss, Israeli, and Dutch health policy arenas all reflect, in different degrees, features of "neocorporatist" policy-making, where governments share the responsibility for social policy with organized interest groups (Lijphart, 1968). New Zealand has a legacy of "Westminster" politics, where traditionally one party had the majority and could play "winner takes all" politics. But, in recent years, the country has experimented with new, regional models of administration. Of the six cases in this study, Singapore appears least bounded by ideology or labels, preferring a pragmatic approach.

Another important point to note is that "styles of governance" are not identical to policy outcomes, though underlying values and dominant orientations make certain policy outcomes more likely than others. Thus values affect policy; conversely, policies may help to reshape and strengthen values (Hirschman, 1970; Marmor, Latham, and Okma, 2006). For example, the British NHS and Canada's Medicare have become important symbols of solidarity in the UK and Canada, and in both countries politicians do not want to be seen undermining the universal coverage.

Theories of historical institutionalism and path dependency (Immergut, 1992; Pierson, 1999; Baumgardner and Jones, 1993) emphasize that major change in social policy is rare; it occurs only in specific circumstances. Institutional legacies and popular support for existing policy arrangements create powerful barriers to change. In this regard, the countries studied in this volume are somewhat atypical: all of them did actually implement major adjustments in the funding, contracting, provision and administration (or governance) of health care. All faced unique "windows of opportunity" for change (Kingdon, 1984). Such opportunities occur, Kingdon argues, at the confluence of three more or less independent streams: the *problem stream* (a general sense of urgency or feeling that a major problem requires action), the *policies stream* (the availability of acceptable and feasible policy solutions based on the gradual accumulation of knowledge and perspectives among specialists), and the *politics stream* (fueled by certain political events, such as a change of administration). Policy entrepreneurs, Kingdon adds, are like surfers waiting for the next big wave (Kingdon, 1984) and the policy window is the opportunity to push their pet solutions. Like a wave, the policy window may disappear again, and thus timing is crucial for presenting and implementing major policy change.

With a similar but somewhat more elaborate approach, Tuohy (1999) has distinguished between a "structural dimension" and an "institutional dimension" of health care systems. The structural dimension reflects the "balance of power" between the three main groups of actors in health care: the state, medical professionals, and private finance. The institutional dimension refers to mechanisms of hierarchy, collegiality, and markets. A major change in the balance of power between the three main groups of actors in health care requires an "extraordinary mobilization of political authority and will" (Tuohy, 1999). Both Taiwan and Singapore provide examples of determined political leaders rapidly implementing reforms by playing crucial roles as policy entrepreneurs.

One theoretical approach used in this volume analyzes the changing behavior of the actors in the health policy arena, including governments, patients, providers, and insurers. Hirschman's notions of "voice" and "exit" are useful tools for analyzing the consequences of health care reform (Hirschman, 1970, 1980, 1993). He sees two classic mechanisms for consumers and citizens to express dissatisfaction with given arrangements: exit or voice. Exit is the base for consumer sovereignty and plays a crucial role in economic traffic. If consumers do not like the price–quality ratio of a given product (and if there is sufficient competition on the market and, therefore, choice), they may simply exit and look elsewhere, thus forcing companies (or governments) to adjust and improve the quality of their goods and services. However, the signal of exit is somewhat poor in information, since it does not provide management with much information on what is wrong. Moreover, exit is an indirect instrument for expressing dissatisfaction, and customers usually do not have interest in improving the products by their withdrawal, but just in finding a better consumption solution (Hirschman, 2008). The second mechanism, voice, usually plays a larger role in the political arena than in the market because, for many consumers or citizens, the exit option (from a region or community) is costly or difficult to put into practice. Citizens thus use their voice in exercising their citizenship, and different political regimes allow for different degrees of voice for their citizens (in the extreme form, i.e. the military dictatorship, opposing voice is eliminated altogether). Voice is costly, can even be dangerous (such in a repressive political system), and usually requires a number of members to start collective action in order to be efficient. On the one hand, voice is a public good since the cost of it to an individual member exceeds any conceivable individual benefit. On the other hand, voice is more frequently performed by loyal members of an organization who are strongly motivated to step in once quality deterioration has passed a certain threshold (Hirschman, 2008). Hirschman (1970) assumed that there was a tradeoff between the two mechanisms of voice and exit: if the two mechanisms are jointly available, the recourse to exit might diminish the volume and power of voice. However, Hirschman (1993) argued that the two could complement each other. He presented situations where exit mechanisms worked better when consumers could also express their voice, and vice versa.

The authors of this volume have all applied combinations of the above economic and public policy models to describe and analyze the health reform experiences of their country of study.

Main Findings

The main findings of this study confirm that, indeed — and not surprising for scholars of public policy — national *values* (or dominant cultural orientations), *institutions*, and *interests* play an important role in the shaping and outcomes of health policy (see also Klein and Marmor, 2006). The combination of fiscal pressures, demographic shifts, and ideological change led to reassessment of existing arrangements everywhere.

The seemingly common experience in external and internal pressure and the similarity in reform goals and means can easily lead to generalized conclusions of (global) convergence. However, the health politics and health policies of the six countries of this study have not converged in one common direction. While the policy problems, policy goals, and range of policy options considered were strikingly similar, the six countries diverged widely in reform directions and processes of implementation. Each country implemented change within the restraints of existing national institutions and political boundaries. Only a few countries systematically studied experiences abroad in their search for new policy directions but in most cases countries "borrowed" reform notions from others without much reflection.

The cases reveal a remarkable variety in reform activity, ranging from the expansion of the basic sick fund model in Israel, changes in central control and regional governance models in New Zealand, to quasi-privatized schemes in Singapore and The Netherlands, the implementation of a uniform nationwide social health insurance in Taiwan, and universal coverage administered by regulated private insurers within the regionally decentralized health system in Switzerland.

The *timing* and *speed of change* of the health reform processes varied as well. In some countries, notably Taiwan and Singapore, the government was able to implement major change rapidly. Others, facing strong opposition from organized stakeholders, had to adjust, delay, or even abandon part or all of their reform efforts. In several cases, the introduction of market competition went hand in hand with increased government control. The current reality of growing diversity and hybridization (or perhaps, "complexification") of health care arrangements also illustrates that countries or health care systems do not fit easily within common categorizations.

One important finding concerns the level of analysis. The last two decades have seen a proliferation of studies that focus on countries as a whole, and seek to place countries in certain categories. For example, the widely quoted work of Esping-Anderson (1990) uses the term "three worlds of welfare" to distinguish three categories of welfare states: the "liberal welfare state," with frugal levels of income protection and means-tested targeted services; the "social-democratic state," with high levels of income protection and tight central control; and the "functionally decentralized consensual, corporatist state." The last refers to countries where the governments share the responsibility for social policy with organized interests.

Such categorization is based on the assumption that countries share certain features that serve as a base for framing certain patterns of inference, and that can help explain developments and outcomes of their social policy. However, over time, systems have changed shape. In fact, most if not all countries' health care systems have become hybridized by combining elements borrowed from the Bismarckian employment-based income protection schemes with the population-wide model of the British NHS. In some areas (most notably, old age pensions and health care), states have assumed more responsibility for income protection than in other areas (such as housing or education). Countries also combine elements of the "liberal welfare state" with arrangements that are more "social-democratic" in nature. With such hybridization, any effort to place countries in preset categories has become problematic (Goodin *et al.*, 1999). Nevertheless, as we will see, certain styles of policy-making are still visible in certain policy areas, for example in the way governments interact with certain organized interest groups in discussing and implementing change in health care.

However, at the level of specific programs and policies, rather than at the national level, we see more similarity in experiences. Most if not all countries are changing the payment mode for hospital care from general budgets based on historical costs to per diem payment, and next, to case-based payment. Almost all countries are moving toward mixed payment models for independent practitioners that combine fees for service with some forms of capitation and specific payment for certain services. Countries with public funding are experimenting with different forms of "purchaser–provider splits" that separate the responsibility for funding health care from the actual provision of services. And almost everywhere, in spite of market rhetoric and stated policy to reduce the role of the state in health care, governments are using their budget control powers to restrain health care expenditure. As another example of a common policy experience, most governments softened the effects of market competition by imposing restrictions on both health insurers and providers of care. This is an example of "bounded privatization": while aiming to shift risks and decision-making power to nonstate actors, governments preserved their regulatory role by mandating certain entitlements in the coverage of private health insurance, forcing private insurance to accept everyone seeking insurance, or imposing national fee schedules for health services or quality norms for both publicly and privately funded health care. Faced with popular opposition, governments often moderated the effects of patient copayments by exempting certain groups.

References

Baumgardner FR, Jones BD. (1993). *Agendas and Instability in American Politics*. University of Chicago Press, Chicago.

Daschle T, Greenberger S, Lambrew J. (2008). *Critical: What We Can Do About the Health-Care Crisis*. Thomas Dunne, New York.

De Swaan A. (1988). *In Care of the State: Health Care, Education and Welfare in Europe and the USA in the Modern Age*. Unity, Oxford.

Douglas M, Wildavsky A. (1982). *Risk and Culture*. University of California Press, Berkeley.

Enthoven AC, Van de Ven WPMM. (2007). "Going Dutch — Managed-competition health insurance in The Netherlands." *New Eng J Med* **357**(24): 2421–2426.

Esping-Anderson G. (1990). *The Three Worlds of Welfare Capitalism*. Polity Press, Cambridge.

Goodin R, Headey B, Muffels R, Dirven H-J. (1999). *The Real Worlds of Welfare Capitalism*. Cambridge University Press, Cambridge.

Hacker JS, Marmor TR. (2007). "How not to think about 'Managed Care.'" In: Marmor TR. (ed.), *Fads, Fallacies and Foolishness in Medical Care Management and Policy*, World Scientific, Singapore.

Harris G. (2007). "Looking at the Dutch and Swiss health systems." *The New York Times*, 30 October.

Helderman J-K. (2007). "Institutional complementarity in Dutch health care reforms: Going beyond the pre-occupation with choice." European Health Policy Group, Berlin, 19–20 April.

Herzlinger RE, Parsa-Parsi R. (2004). "Consumer-driven health care." *J Am Med Assoc* **292**(10): 1213–1220.

Hirschman AO. (1970). *Exit, Voice and Loyalty: Responses to Decline in Firms, Organizations, and States*. Harvard University Press, Cambridge.

Hirschman AO. (1980). "'Exit, voice, and loyalty': Further reflections and a survey of recent contributions." *Health Soc* **58**(3): 430–453.

Hirschman AO. (1993). "Exit, voice and the fate of the German democratic republic: An essay in conceptual history." *World Polit* **45**(2): 173–202.

Hirschman AO. (2008). "Exit and voice." In: Durlauf S, Basingstoke BL (eds.), *The Palgrave Dictionary of Economics*, 2nd ed. Palgrave Macmillan, New York.

Immergut EM. (1992). *Health Politics: Interests and Institutions in Western Europe*. Cambridge University Press, Cambridge.

Kingdon J. (1984). *Agendas, Alternatives, and Public Policies.* Longman, New York.

Klein R. (1995). *Learning From Others: Shall the Last Be the First Markets?* Four Country Conference on Health Care Policies and Health Care Reforms in the United States, Canada, Germany and The Netherlands. Amsterdam, 23–25 February, Ministry of Health, Welfare and Sport, The Hague.

Klein R. (2006). *The New Politics of the NHS*, 5th ed. Longman Group, Harlow.

Klein R, Marmor TR. (2006). "Reflections on Policy Analysis: Putting It Together Again." In *The Oxford Handbook of Political Science.* Oxford University Press, Oxford.

Labra ME. (2007). Notas Críticas Sobre Estatificación Socioeconómica, Copagos y Acceso en los Servicios Públicos de Salud de Chile. *Revista Española de Economía de la Salud* **6**(1): 46–50.

Lasswell H. (1985). *Politics: Who Gets What, When, How*, 2nd ed. World, Cleveland.

Leu RE, Rutten FH, Brouwer W, Matter P, Ruetschi C. (2009). *The Swiss and Dutch Health Insurance Systems: Universal Coverage and Regulated Competitive Markets.* The Commonwealth Fund, New York.

Lijphart A. (1968). *Verzuiling, Pacificatie en Kengtering in de Nederlandse Politiek* ("Pillarization, Pacification and Change in Dutch Politics"). JH de Bussy, Amsterdam.

Maarse H, Okma KGH. (2004). "The Privatisation Paradox in Dutch Health Care." In: Maarse H (ed.), *Privatisation in European Health Care.* Elsevier Gezondheidszorg, Maarssen.

Marmor TR. (1998). "Hype and Hyperbole: The rhetoric and realities of managerial reform in health care." *J Health Serv Res Policy* **3**(1): 62–64.

Marmor TR, Okma KGH. (2003). "Health care systems in transition, by the World Health Organization." *J Health Polit Policy Law* **28**(4): 747–755.

Marmor TR, Mashaw JL, Harvey PL, eds. (1990). *America's Misunderstood Welfare State, Persisting Myths, Enduring Realities.* Basic, New York.

Marmor TR, Okma KGH, Lathan SR. (2006). "Values, institutions and health politics. Comparative perspectives." In: Wendt C, Wolf C (eds.), *Soziologie der Gesundheit. Kolner Zeitschrift fur Soziologie und Sozialpsychologie.* Special volume **46**: 383–405.

Marmor TR, Freeman R, Okma KGH. (2005). "Comparative perspectives and policy learning in the world of health care." *J Compar Policy Anal* **7**(4): 331–348.

Ministerie van Volksgezondheid, Welzijn en Sport (2008). Accessed 20 October 2008. http://www.minvws.nl.

Naik G. (2007). "Dutch treatment: In Holland, some see model for US health care system." *Wall St J* 6 Sep.

OECD. (1992). *The Reform of Health Care: A Comparative Analysis of Seven OECD Countries. Health Reform Studies No. 2.* OECD, Paris.

OECD. (1994). *The Reform of Health Care: A Review of Seventeen OECD Countries. Health Reform Studies No. 5.* OECD, Paris.

OECD (2006). *Review of Health Systems: Switzerland.* OECD, Paris.

Okma KGH. (1997). *Studies in Dutch Health Politics, Policies and Law.* Ph.D. thesis. University of Utrecht.

Okma KGH. (1999). "Review of European health care reform: Analysis of current strategies, by Richard B. Saltman and Josep Figueras." *J Health Polit Policy Law* **24**(4): 835–840.

Okma KGH. (2002). "What is the best public–private model for Canadian health care?" *Policy Matters* **3**(6). Canadian Institute for Research on Public Policy, Montreal.

Okma KGH, De Roo AA (forthcoming). "From Polder Model to modern management in Dutch health care." In: Marmor TR, Freeman R, Okma KGH (eds.), *Comparative Studies and The Politics of Modern Medical Care.* Yale University Press, New Haven.

Palmer, GR, Short SD. (1989). *Health Care and Public Policy — An Australian Analysis.* The Macmillan Company of Australia, Melbourne.

Pierson P. (1994). *Dismantling the Welfare State: Reagan, Thatcher and the Politics of Retrenchment.* Cambridge University Press, Cambridge.

Pickard S, Sheaff R, Dowling B. (2006). "Exit, voice, governance and user-responsiveness: The case of English primary care trusts." *Soc Sci Med* **63**(1): 373–383.

Ranade W, ed. (1998). *Markets and Health Care: A Comparative Analysis.* Addison-Wesley Longman, New York.

Reinhardt UE. (2004). "The Swiss health system. Regulated competition without managed care." *J Am Med Assoc* **292**(10): 1227–1231.

Timmins N. (1995). *The Five Giants: A Biography of the Welfare State*. Fontana, London.

Tuohy CH. (1993). "Social policy: Two worlds." In: Atkinson M (ed.), *Governing Canada, Institutions and Public Policy*. Harcourt Brace Canada, Toronto.

Tuohy CH. (1999). *Accidental Logics: The Dynamics of Change in the Health Care Arena in the United States, Britain, and Canada*. Oxford University Press, New York.

Van de Ven WPMM, Schut FT. (2008). "Universal mandatory health insurance in The Netherlands: A model for the United States?" *Health Affairs* **27**(3): 771–781.

Wilensky HL. (2002). *Rich Democracies, Political Economy, Public Policy, and Performance*. University of California Press, Berkeley.

World Bank. (2006). *World Development Indicators 2006*. The World Bank, Washington. World Health Organization (2008). Accessed 27 Dec. 2008. www.who.org.

Israel: Partial Health Care Reform as Laboratory of Ongoing Change

David Chinitz*,† *and Rachel Meislin*‡

Historical Background

Israel, a small country of seven million inhabitants on the eastern shore of the Mediterranean, bordered by Lebanon, Jordan, and Egypt, is another country with a long tradition of public health insurance. But even 60 years after the creation of the State of Israel, analysts of current trends in the country's geopolitics and political economy highlight the impact of the institutions that were in place while the State was "in waiting."

The General Sick Fund (GSF) and the Histadrut Labor Federation were among the most important structures. At the time of Israel's major health reform, the enactment of the National Health Insurance Law in 1995, the Labor Union Histadrut owned the GSF. However, historically, the latter preceded the former: the GSF was formed in 1912, while the Labor Federation was established some years later (Chinitz, 1995; Ellencweig, 1983). This is one of several examples in which (health) solidarity arrangements have risen from the grassroots, to be later taken over or managed by higher governing entities. From the outset, this dynamic has created tensions between civil society and government in the health policy realm.

* Corresponding author.
† Braun School of Public Health, The Hebrew University-Hadassah, Jerusalem. Email: chinitz@cc.huji.ac.il.
‡ Department of Health Policy and Management, School of Public Health, Hebrew University-Hadassah, Jerusalem.

After the creation of the State of Israel, different stakeholders harbored different assumptions about the fate of the pre-State institutions. Israel's first Prime Minister, David Ben Gurion, envisioned that the new apparatus of the State would encompass the activities of the pre-State institutions, rendering them superfluous (Chinitz, 1995). Decades of existence of these institutions had created strong path dependency, limiting the expansion of government sovereignty. In a number of areas, Israel's governing apparatus featured competing giants — government on the one hand, and ongoing civil society institutions of the pre-State era on the other — contending for control over the activities of the new State. This tension helps explain Israel's particular styles of health governance today (elements of corporatist bargaining combined with strong state control), and its attitudes towards exit, voice, loyalty, and their corollary: accountability. Traditionally, the assignment of responsibility for finance and provision of health services has been unclear, nested within an ownership structure that has many blurred lines. Thus, Israel's accountability for the financial and service outcomes of public services remains weak. Indeed, the modern Hebrew language has no widely accepted word for "accountability."

The sick funds that existed at the time of the creation of the State originally numbered eight; the number then dropped to four. All had political ties, and some had tight relationships with other civic organizations. The GSF, for example, had enrolled 80% of the population by the early 1980s (while 15% of the population had enrolled with one of the three smaller funds). At that time, it had strong ties with both the Labor Federation and the Labor Party, which ran Israel's governing coalition from 1948 to 1977 (Ellencweig, 1983). This iron triangle (Labor Federation, Labor Party, and the GSF) created a situation in which the GSF competed with the Ministry of Health for dominance. Both the GSF and the Ministry of Health engaged in planning and operating health services. The GSF was able to use its political leverage and close ties to the Labor Federation and Labor Party to escape accountability for deficit spending on expanding health services. In turn, the GSF was beholden to the Labor Federation, and obligated to enroll any of the latter's members. Indeed, Labor Federation members and employees were automatically enrolled in the GSF (the

Labor Federation had signed up 60% of the country's labor force during the first two-and-a-half decades of the State's existence). The GSF thus had a captive membership and relatively little incentive to be responsive to members' needs and wants. Since the GSF could count on friendly government aid, it did not need to worry about the makeup of its membership.

In the late 1980s, 95% of the population had voluntarily enrolled with one of the four not-for-profit funds. Despite this nearly universal coverage, the system was plagued by financial instability, public and provider dissatisfaction, hospital overcapacity, and fragmentation of services (Chinitz, 1995; Penchas and Shani, 1995). In addition — at least in the eyes of the Israeli public and Israeli politicians — there were too many uninsured.[1]

Forces Leading to Reform

External forces eventually prompted the government to act. In 1977, the Labor Party's arch-competitor, the Herut Party, unseated Labor and became the leader of the new governing coalition. Herut's successor, Likud, remained in power until the early 1990s, sometimes in unity governments with Labor. With Likud in power, the rules of the game changed for the GSF and the Histadrut. With a policy agenda that aimed, in part, to dismantle the iron triangle, Likud reduced government subsidies in areas like health care, tried to limit the autonomy of the GSF, and promoted some of the smaller sick funds, like the Maccabi Sick Fund, by capitalizing on the increasing perception that the GSF represented the bureaucratic ways of the past (Rosen and Bennun, 2007). Moreover, the Maccabi Sick Fund offered its members greater freedom in choosing their physicians, a vast improvement over the GSF's practice. Younger and wealthier (and healthier) populations began to desert the GSF and enroll in Maccabi, and, arguably, the

---

[1] As in The Netherlands, even a small share of uninsured can create enough political pressure for the government to take action. This idea will be expanded on further in coming sections.

notion of "exit" (Hirschman, 1970) came into play for the first time in Israeli health care history. As contributions (both member fees and employer contributions) for health insurance were based on income as earmarked taxes, Maccabi built up higher revenues and could therefore offer lower member contributions than its competitors. In the 1980s, a two-tier health system became an issue of much public debate, and eventually became palpable to Israeli society.

When the Knesset passed the National Health Insurance Law in 1994, it was largely due to a confluence of the above factors. Other factors also contributed to the climate for change: increased consumerism, the weakening of the Histadrut and its ties with the Labor Party (some of whose members began to view the Labor Federation and the GSF as a burden rather than a boon), and the influence of the worldwide trend towards "reinventing government." Moreover, citizens were dissatisfied with their providers' lack of responsiveness and long waiting times (especially for GSF members), there was a pervasive public perception of inequality in the health care system (including the arbitrary bureaucratic rules regarding the rights of sick fund members), and health professionals (including Ministry of Health employees) were increasing their technocratic knowhow. In passing a socially progressive universal health insurance law emphasizing patient choice, the health system was Israel's change leader. In other areas, like education, change was hampered by the pre-State heritage of pluralism, weak regulatory capacity, and weak accountability for budgets and performance.

The 1995 National Health Insurance Law (NHI) mandates all residents to register with a sick fund (similar to the mandates of the Swiss and Dutch health insurances; see the chapters on Switzerland and The Netherlands). The NHI is a population-wide social health insurance, administered by four major competing sick funds. It was part of a three-pronged reform proposed in 1990 by the Netanyahu Commission, a state commission of inquiry (Rosen, 2003). The two other planks of the reform — transforming government hospitals into public trusts and the reorganization of the Ministry of Health — never materialized. Those proposals faced too much resistance from hospital labor unions and stakeholders unwilling to commit the necessary financing for transferring services from the Health Ministry's budget to the sick funds.

From a rational planning point of view, the partial implementation of the reform is a recipe for frustration. Nonetheless, from a policy-learning point of view, the NHI's enactment set in motion a chain of events worth examining (Helderman *et al.*, 2005). The enactment led to one radical change that in itself did not depend on the full implementation of the envisioned reform: a legally defined universal standard basket of services. Previously, each fund could determine its own entitlements, and was not required to provide any particular service. While other countries like The Netherlands (Berg, Van der Grinten, and Klazinga, 2004) and New Zealand (Chinitz, 1999) abandoned the idea of (explicitly) defining a core basket of health services, Israel went quite clearly, if not always resolutely, down this road.

Funding and Providing Health Care in Israel

The major funding sources for health care in Israel are social insurance contributions, tax subsidy, and modest amounts of patient copayments (Rosen, 2003). In recent years, copayments for prescription drugs have increased, but there are many exemptions and caps on the total amount which families have to pay each year, with lower caps for the elderly (Rosen, 2003). While the mandatory social health insurance offers a wide range of entitlements, supplemental health insurance plays a marginal (but growing) role (see below). It offers coverage for the costs of private physicians, treatment in private clinics, and complementary medicine.

Israelis can choose the fund they want to register with, and can change it four times per year. In 1995, the first year that Israelis had this option, about 4% of the population switched funds, but after that the rate of change decreased to about 1%. The largest fund, Clalit, covers just over 50% of the population. The NHI explicitly lists its entitlements. It not only specifies procedures and pharmaceuticals covered, but also provides guidelines for applications. If a physician prescribes an "outside of the guideline" use of a particular drug, the sick fund is within its legal rights to refuse to reimburse.[2] Parliament can add (or delist) entitlements within the available public budget to cover the anticipated costs (the Ministry of Finance agreed to increase the annual budget by about 1% for this expansion). In 1998, the government set up a Public Committee to assess the addition of new services (Chinitz *et al.*, 1998). The Committee meets several times a year and the media regularly cover its activities. It ranks potential new services by way of a health technology assessment, provided by the Ministry of Health (MoH). In a somewhat neocorporatist mode, the 24-person Committee is made up of physicians, public representatives, and experts from the MoH and the sick funds (Rosen, 2003). The Committee decides which services will be included based on ethical, economic, and social criteria. Not surprisingly, the list of services seeking entrance to the basket, mainly pharmaceuticals, usually exceeds the available funding, and there is much pressure from patients and lobby groups to expand the entitlements.

The insured can seek supplementary insurance offered both by sick funds and by private health insurance (about 34% of the population chose the latter, but this share has not increased in recent years) (Gross *et al.*, 2007). In recent years, some funds have expanded their supplemental coverage with prescription drugs and other services not covered under the basic insurance. Ironically, the Ministry of Finance opposed this move, as it would increase national health expenditure and create a two-tiered system. The result of this debate (see below) was to curtail supplemental insurance coverage while expanding the budget for the standard basket.

Health care services include hospitals owned by the government and sick funds, clinics owned by sick funds, self-employed physicians who have contracts with funds, and private for-profit hospitals, laboratories, and institutional care. Mother-and-child care (including prenatal care, vaccinations in the first year of life, and developmental monitoring until school age), mental health care, and nursing care are not included in the

---

[2] Qualitative research by Chinitz indicates that Israeli physicians spend up to 10% of their time engaged in quarrels with sick fund managers over these points. The physicians often win the argument, but the organizational consequences in terms of efficiency and morale are significant.

NHI and are subject to different arrangements. All insured can select a primary care physician who works in their health fund's clinic, or a self-employed physician who has a contract with their fund. Access to non-emergency care generally requires a referral from the health fund physician or preapproval from the fund. While Israelis can, and do, exercise choice of hospital, referrals generally specify a particular provider. Hospitals receive capped budgets, though the funds typically reimburse 50% of budget overruns. Emergency care and outpatient clinics are paid on a fee-for-service basis. Physicians usually receive salaries, often combined with a capitation payment for each patient on their list. Independent physicians receive a capitation payment for their patients. The capitation payments are generally a form of capped fee-for-service, as physicians do not receive additional payment for follow-up visits; the physicians payments do not face financial risks for prescriptions and referrals. The MoH sets the per diem rates and fee schedules for the entire country.

National professional associations of hospital physicians, nurses, and other providers negotiate salaries on behalf of their members. In Jerusalem, physicians are permitted private work in hospitals under strict regulation. Elsewhere, ad hoc arrangements allowed physicians to do private work in hospitals, but they were halted by order of the State Attorney General and the issue has not yet been resolved. Many physicians based in public hospitals have after-hours private practices and perform procedures at private hospitals. The collective bargaining and active participation of the main organized stakeholders resembles the neocorporatist style of social policy-making in Western Europe. In general, this arrangement gives providers of care strong veto position.

The sick funds are legally independent entities, but the MoH is responsible overall. It sets the rules, defines benefits, is involved in the planning and allocation of budgets, sets hospital budgets, and imposes limits on public spending as well as on the number of physicians. The National Health Insurance Institute administers the funding of the NHI. It collects contributions via the tax system and provides funding to the sick funds.

The MoH has monitored both the basic insurance and supplemental coverage. Private insurers can set their own premiums, and membership is subject to underwriting, similar to the supplemental health insurance in The Netherlands. The National Health Insurance Regulator (or Insurance Regulator), a branch of the Ministry of Finance, regulates private health insurance. Recently, the Insurance Regulator intervened and overturned private insurers' refusal to pay for pharmaceuticals for which a substitute existed in the national standard basket of services.

While the MoH has strengthened its oversight of the sick funds since the enactment of the NHI, it has the reputation of being a somewhat ineffective regulator. Part of this reputation results from the fact that the MoH owns two-thirds of general hospital beds. This has created a conflict of interest and sometimes an inability to turn its attention from the day-to-day management of hospitals towards planning and regulation. In recent years, the MoH has turned out to be better at financial regulation than at quality assurance, though it has taken strides in the latter realm as well. Through control over hospital reimbursement rates, the MoH has been able to stabilize health expenditure. As of 2006, the health funds were, by and large, working within balanced budgets for the standard basket of services. The Ministry has been less effective at regulating quality of care. Lacking resources and confronting less-than-complete cooperation from physicians' associations, it has not been able to create a framework for ongoing quality assurance in provision and insurance. Physicians' associations and health funds participate in benchmarking and other quality assurance efforts, but have not agreed on public disclosure of measured results. The MoH is a frequent target of critical media coverage in the event of medical error and malfeasance, and has set up investigative and disciplinary committees to deal with these concerns.

Israeli health policy-making thus provides an interesting example of strong government involvement on one hand and political timidity in enacting radical change on the other. The strong veto position of organized interests evidently contributes to the government's incapacity to implement change rapidly. But the Israeli experience may also be illustrative of another phenomenon: that partially implemented reforms may offer a more realistic and interesting comparative experience than "perfect" policy reform that is not implemented.

Results, Failures, and Continuing Evolution of the Health Insurance Reform of 1995

The 1995 NHI law improved the regulation of the existing sick funds that already covered 95% of the population. The preamble to the law states that it aims to provide "justice, equity, and mutual aid." The main provision is the requirement that all residents take out health insurance coverage with one of the four sick funds. There are open enrollments, and the insured can switch funds each year. The insured pay income-related contributions to the National Insurance Institute (these contributions replaced the former membership dues paid directly to the sick funds). The NHI established a standard basket of services that all sick funds must provide. It also calculated the cost of the standard basket, as a base for determining the overall budget for the system. The government covers any gap between revenue and prospective expenditure for the basket. The National Insurance Institute allocates the available funds to the sick funds through a capitation formula weighted only for age (an interesting difference from the complicated formula in the Dutch sick fund budget model; see the chapter on The Netherlands).

The NHI was one of three prongs of the health reform proposed by the Judicial State Commission of Inquiry in 1990. While it dealt mainly with finance and rights to health care, the other two prongs of the report proposed reforming the administration of hospitals and modernizing the MoH. Government-owned hospitals were to become trusts, and mental health care and long-term care services provided directly by the Ministry were to transfer to the sick fund basket. These two planks were never fully implemented. However, the establishment of the NHI led to important changes in the financial relationship between sick funds and hospitals, and at the beginning of the 21st century there are new attempts to transfer the responsibility for mental health care to the sick funds (see below).

Notwithstanding this "reform shortfall," change vectors inevitably continue to influence the system. During the 13 years since the NHI's inception, new forces of change have emerged, some — no surprise — as a result of the implementation of the law itself. What is striking about the Israeli health system case is that one can identify significant areas of policy learning in which the basic parameters of the system survive and adapt to challenges. In other words, the subsequent incremental changes that have occurred after the NHI's enactment have, to some degree, played out in ways that do not appear to have been intended by the major stakeholders. The section below describes some of the major innovations that have been evolving incrementally in the system.

Determining the Health Care Entitlements of Israel's Social Insurance

The NHI updates the standard basket of services almost every year; in some years the Ministry of Finance provides little or no funding for expanding the coverage. The expansion (mainly prescription drugs) to the basket is based on the recommendations of an expert panel consisting of representatives of the MoH, sick fund, and physicians' associations, as well as public figures, ethicists, and economists. The MoH's Health Technology Unit provides its assessments to the committee based on reviews of the literature regarding the cost-effectiveness of interventions and the number of patients affected. At one time, high-profile pressure exerted by patients' groups (such as colon cancer patients conducting a hunger strike in an effort to get the prescription drug Avastin included in the benefit basket) was an effective strategy. But recently these efforts have become less and less effective. It appears that the Israeli public and policy-makers have started to accept this sad truth: not all drugs that might benefit patients can be funded.

However, the NHI permits sick funds to offer supplemental insurance for services not included in the standard basket. Supplemental plans face procompetitive regulation that prohibits underwriting, and insurers have to set community-rated flat rate premiums by age group. Though the sick funds initially offered supplemental policies as a marketing device, they recently became a strategic tool in budgetary negotiations with the Ministry of Finance. When the Ministry of Finance did not provide additional funds for updating the standard basket in the 2007 budget cycle, Macabbi and the GSF offered additional supplemental insurance that would cover the "life-saving" drugs not included in the standard basket. The Ministry of Finance opposed these expanded supplemental policies on the grounds of inequity and loss of control over national health expenditure. So, though the MoH at first supported the supplemental policies, it agreed to roll them back when the Ministry of Finance increased the available budget to update the standard basket and include the life-saving drugs. How the MoH will define "life-saving" in the future, however, remains to be seen, and supplemental policies may continue to grow.

Patients' Rights

The Knesset passed the Patients' Rights Law in 1996, soon after the NHI. The law defines and regulates the relationship between patient and health care provider. It views the patient as an autonomous actor in the health care system with rights to quality, privacy, and professionalism. The law includes provisions like the right to a second opinion, informed consent, and medical confidentiality. It also established patients' rights representatives within the hospital setting, and ethics, inspection, and quality control committees. The matter of patients' rights seems to be more of an issue in care settings, especially hospitals, than in the context of sick fund member relations.

All sick funds and hospitals have developed electronic patient records (EPRs) which aim to improve the appropriateness, coordination, and continuity of care. However, the EPRs differ within each constituent of the system. There is no standard data model and often more than one type of model per hospital, even while one study has reported that physicians do work with EMRs in over 98% of departments (Lejbkowicz, 2004).

However, as in other countries, unifying the data sets becomes challenging as issues regarding privacy emerge.

Financing

The significant changes in market share among the sick funds that occurred in the years before and the two years after the NHI's enactment have tapered off; currently, only about 1% of the population switches funds every year (Shmueli, 2007). Perhaps the low number of transfers is to be expected with no price competition over the standard basket, and with registration located in post offices where the sick funds cannot easily engage in risk selection. A reasonable assessment is that the sick fund market is "contestable," meaning that sick funds try to avoid losing members, even if their reputation and marketing efforts are not likely to expand their market share.

As noted above, the sick funds receive their budget based on a capitation formula weighted only for age (Rosen, 2003; Shmueli *et al.*, 2007). Despite the fact that the capitation formula is not adjusted for health status within age groups, there do not seem to be signs of significant quality skimping, such as undertreating chronically ill patients. Still, some argue that the funds can influence selection based on which services they offer (Rosen, 2003), and analysis of the small percentage of individuals moving among funds cannot rule out quality skimping (Shmueli, 2007).

While the sick funds shy away from alienating members by restricting free choice of provider, there is some channeling of patients to preferred providers in the spirit of selective contracting. One incentive for this behavior is the "capping" of hospital budgets. Under this arrangement, regulated by the MoH, each sick fund pays every general hospital a combination of DGR, fee-for-service, and per diem payment. Based on estimates of expected use, each sick fund pays full price up to a budget cap, with a 50% discount above the cap. The sick funds thus have an incentive to channel patients to hospitals that have exceeded the cap (Rosen, 2003). It does not appear that choice is a salient issue with patients, however, as they can insist on going to the hospital of their choice. However, one major hospital and the GSF went public with their dispute over payment negotiations and issues concerning the cap and freedom to channel patients. In the end they reached a compromise: the MoH has announced legislation to guarantee patients with certain diseases (mainly cancer) free choice of hospital.

Since 1998, as part of the annual Omnibus Budget Arrangement Act initiated by the Ministry of Finance, sick funds have been able to seek approval for copayments (Brammli-Greenberg *et al.*, 2006). Research has shown that in 2007, 12% of the population did forego consuming health services and goods, especially pharmaceuticals, presumably due to the cost of copayments. Among low-income patients, 20% desisted from using the same health services due to cost in 2007, an impressive decrease from 30% in 2005 (Gross *et al.*, 2007).

Access and Equity

While inequity in access to health care has undoubtedly decreased since the NHI, health inequality has become a focus of concern. At least one sick fund has initiated a program aimed at closing gaps among its members in terms of access to care, primary prevention, and cultural competency (Epstein *et al.*, 2006). Problems still exist among minority populations. One study discovered that among the members of Clalit, the biggest sick fund, Israeli Arabs are much less likely to utilize medical services, although they are insured under the same terms (Shmueli, 2000).

The sick funds have also recently focused on quality of care. Under the auspices of the MoH and in conjunction with a health services research group, the sick funds are collaborating in developing benchmarks for standards of care in the community setting. These benchmarks are not binding, however, and it is up to each fund how to use the measures and publicize its own activities. It is important to note that the collaboration in such quality assurance activities expresses a certain consensus over the validity of evidence-based medicine.

In 2006, the MoH and the Ministry of Finance agreed to transfer mental health care services from the former to the sick funds. However, as of late 2008, the necessary legislation has passed only the first of three readings in Parliament and the planned reform is currently being discussed by a parliamentary subcommittee (Chinitz, 2009; Aviram and Ginath, 2006). Controversy persists over whether such a transfer constitutes privatization of the service, whether the sick funds will provide quality services in this realm, and the future of those currently employed in the government system.

The two sick funds that had been dominated by labor union affiliations in their governing boards have seen these arrangements altered to reduce the role of the unions. The question of who governs the sick funds arises in various contexts periodically, for example in high-profile coverage of sick fund management's large salaries. Focus on these matters indicates the persisting difficulty in defining lines of ownership, control, and accountability in the health system.

Theoretical Implications of the Israeli Case: The Role of the State and the Dominant Cultural Orientation

The picture painted above is one of major reform in the health insurance realm, stalled reform or incremental change in other aspects of the system, and policy learning in both. Regarding the role of the state, it appears that the Ministry of Finance, while trying to restrain public and national health expenditure, has also become accountable for perceptions that the health system is underfunded (despite budgetary increases) and becoming increasingly financially privatized. The MoH, while trying to strengthen its own role as a regulator, is still occupied with provision of services and ownership of hospitals.

In terms of the dominant cultural orientation, it appears that underlying values of social solidarity in health care remain. Key stakeholders criticize every move they perceive as privatization, because it could potentially introduce inequity into the system. Hirschman's notions of exit, voice, and loyalty (1970) form a worthy theoretical framework through which one may view the progression of the Israeli health care system. While the main thrust of reforms has been oriented towards competition, namely exit, the ongoing debates regarding health care indicate that "voice" is very much at work in maintaining accountability among the constituents of the system. Most Israelis, both policy-makers and the public, consider voice of great value to the system. In fact, researchers recently consulted directly the public on four issues of equity in health care, and on prioritizing the medications and treatments available through the health basket. One hundred and thirty-two randomly sampled individuals participated in a "Health Parliament," in an effort to seek consensus on these issues (Guttman *et al.*, 2008). Summaries of the citizens' responses were sent to the Minister of Health and to the public committee that updates the standard basket of services. While the results of the Health Parliament were apparently of interest to the members of decision-making bodies, the activity was not continued, for budgetary reasons.

Choice is a value, too, and seems not to be limited by selective contracting to any great degree. But exit seems almost insignificant as a mechanism of accountability in the system. Small countries like Israel or The Netherlands do not really offer many exit options to any one party in the system. Notwithstanding the low levels of actual exit, however, the threat of exit may exert pressure on sick funds and providers to improve service, and may also enhance the role of voice (Chinitz, 2000).

Overall, it could be argued that the Israeli health system has evolved in terms of increased financial accountability and maintenance of a broad range of entitlements subject to explicit rationing of new technologies. It also offers interesting opportunities for policy learning in areas like quality assurance and contracting between payers and providers. However, the role of the MoH is still impacted by the blurred lines of authority and responsibility that date back to the early formation of the Israeli political economy and social systems. Path dependency has been most strongly felt in regard to the role of the MoH, and its ability to regulate the system has been disadvantaged as a result. Even so, incremental learning is occurring in regard to quality assurance, patient records, and perhaps even mental health reform. One could say that Israel is on the cusp of finding a viable balance between exit, voice, and choice, but for reasons dating back to the origins of the dominant cultural orientations in the society, actors tend to fall back into patterns of unclear assignment of authority and responsibility.

References

Aviram U, Ginath Y, eds. (2006). *Mental Health Services in Israel: Trends and Issues.* Cherikover, Tel-Aviv.

Berg M, Van der Grinten T, Klazinga N. (2004). "Technology Assessment, Priority Setting, and Appropriate Care in Dutch Health Care." *Int J Tech Assess Health Care* **20**(1): 35–43.

Brammli-Greenberg S, Rosen B, Gross R. (2006). *Co-payments for Physician Visits: How Large Is the Burden and Who Bears the Brunt?* Jerusalem: Myers-JDC-Brookdale Institute.

Chinitz D. (1995). "Israel's Health Policy Breakthrough: The Politics of Reform and the Reform of Politics." *J Health Polit Policy Law* **20**(4): 909–932.

Chinitz D. (1999). "Israel's Basic Basket of Health Services; Technocracy vs. Democracy Revisited." *Soc Security* **54**: 53–68.

Chinitz D. (2000). "Regulated Competition and Citizen Participation: Lessons from Israel." *Health Expectations* **3**(2): 90–96.

Chinitz D, Shalev C, Galai N, Israeli A. (1998). "Israel's Basic Basket of Services: The Importance of Being Explicitly Implicit." *BMJ* **317**: 1005–1007.

Ellencweig A. (1983). "The New Israeli Health Care Reform: An Analysis of a National Need." *J Health Polit Policy Law* **8**(2): 366–386.

Epstein L *et al.* (2006). *Reducing Health Inequality and Health Inequity in Israel: Towards a National Policy and Action Program — Summary Report.* The Smokler Center for Health Policy Research, Myers-JDC-Brookdale Institute, Jerusalem.

Gross R, Brammli-Greenberg S, Matzliach R. (2007). *Public Opinion on the Level of Service and Performance of the Health Care System Ten Years after the Introduction of National Health Insurance.* Myers-JDC-Brookdale Institute, Jerusalem.

Guttman N *et al.* (2008). "What Should Be Given Priority — Costly Medications for Relatively Few People or Inexpensive Ones for Many? The Health Parliament Public Consultation Initiative in Israel." *Health Expectations* **11**: 177–188.

Helderman J-K, Schut FT. Van der Grinten TED, Van de Ven WPMM. (2005). "Market-Oriented Health Care Reforms and Policy Learning in the Netherlands." *J Health Polit Policy Law* **30**(1–2): 189–210.

Hirschman AO. (1970). *Exit, Voice, and Loyalty: Responses to Declines in Firms, Organizations, and States.* Harvard University Press, Cambridge.

Lejbkowicz I, Denekamp Y, Reis S, Goldenberg D. (2004). "Electronic Medical Record Systems in Israel's Public Hospitals." *Israeli Med Assoc J* **6**(10): 583–587.

Penchas S, Shani M. (1995). "Redesigning a National Health-Care System: The Israeli Experience." *Int J Health Care Qual Assur* **8**(2): 9–17.

Rosen B. (2003). *Health Care Systems in Transition: Israel.* European Observatory of Health Care Systems, Copenhagen.

Rosen B, Bennun G. (2007). National Health Insurance: Why in 1994? In: Bennun G, Ofer G (eds.), *Ten Years of National Health Insurance.* Israel Institute for Health Policy Research (Hebrew), Tel Hashomer.

Shmueli A. (2000). "Inequities in Health. Inequality in Medical Care in Israel: Arabs and Jews in the Jerusalem District of the General Sick Fund." *Eur J Pub Health* **10**(1): 18–23.

Shmueli A, Chinitz D. (2001). "Risk-Adjusted Capitation: The Israeli Experience." *Eur J Pub Health* **11**(2): 182–184.

Shmueli A, Bendelac J, Achdut L. (2007). "Who Switches Health Funds in Israel?" *Health Econ Policy Law* **2**(3): 251–265.

Chapter 2

Change and Continuity in Dutch Health Care: Origins and Consequences of the 2006 Health Insurance Reforms[1]

Kieke G. H. Okma and Hans Maarse

Introduction

In 2006, the Dutch government introduced a population-wide health insurance scheme that replaced the former public and private health insurances. With that step, it abolished the sick fund insurance that had covered wage earners and their dependents for over 50 years.[2] The Dutch parliament passed the law in 2005, after surprisingly little political debate or

[1] This chapter, in particular the descriptive part, draws heavily on a contribution by Okma and De Roo, "From Polder Model to Modern Management in Dutch Health Care," for the forthcoming book *Comparative Studies and Modern Medical Care: Learning Opportunity or Global Mythology* (Theodore R. Marmor, Richard Freeman, and Kieke GH. Okma, eds.), to be published by Yale University Press in 2009. That chapter also served as the base for a paper presented by the first author at the Annual Meeting of the National Academy of Social Insurance (NASI), in January 2008 (Okma, 2008).

[2] While there is no generally accepted legal definition of "social insurance," it commonly refers to a particular set of rules imposed by the government: mandatory participation for all or large parts of the population, prepaid contributions that usually are levied as a share of gross income, employers sharing the payments with their employees, and government-determined entitlements. In Germany and other Western European countries, social insurance schemes allocated the administrative responsibility to sick funds (or "sickness funds") that already existed as mutual income protection schemes. In a way, those 19th century sick funds played a role as organized consumer groups that contracted health services on behalf of their members.

public opposition. In essence, the new insurance scheme is similar to earlier proposals of the 1980s and 1990s that failed to gain lasting public and political support after partial implementation. But the new law meant a further push towards privatization of Dutch health insurance and health care.

Foreign as well as national commentators and policy-makers have hailed the Dutch model as a triumph of consumerism and an example for other countries. Likewise, Enthoven and Van de Ven (2007) suggest that the U.S. might want to copy the Dutch model. A lengthy front-page article in *The Wall Street Journal* enthusiastically embraces "Holland as Model for U.S. Health Care" (Naik, 2007). *The New York Times* sees the Dutch model (together with that of Switzerland) as a good example for the U.S. as it would "eliminate the role of employers" (Harris, 2007).

What led to the new insurance model in Holland in 2006? What explains the remarkably smooth transition? Does it really represent a dramatic break with the past, heralding a new (and untested) model of social insurance administered by private insurers? Or, perhaps, a private insurance system under public regulation? What has been the role of organized stakeholders in the reform process? How does it work? And what has actually happened after its introduction — and what can be expected to happen in the future?

To answer these questions, this chapter starts with a brief sketch of the development of social and private health insurance in The Netherlands in the 20th century. It addresses some of the particular characteristics of Dutch social policy-making, the core features of the current system, and the history of the 2006 health reform.

The chapter looks at the changing positions of the main stakeholders in Dutch health care, including health care providers and insurers, as well as the government itself. It shows how insurers and providers alike adjusted their attitudes and behavior in reaction to — and in anticipation of — announced health reforms, even when some of that policy was not implemented. And, once such changed behavior became visible and generally accepted, it encouraged governments to change its course and to take up reform proposals that had been rejected a decade before. Dutch patients and consumers, too, faced new options, and have reacted in quite divergent ways, sometimes initiating and supporting change, sometimes forcing the government to reverse its course.

The chapter concludes that rather than a dramatic break with the past, the Dutch health reform represents much continuity in the role of the government and other actors in Dutch health care. The 2006 health insurance scheme replaced the former public and private health insurance, but not the long-term care insurance which remained public. It also did not do away with much of the existing government regulation. As the main stakeholders had already anticipated the reforms, there was a more gradual change than a dramatic break with the past. The new scheme did not so much replace or complement previous governance models as create a complicated "complementarity" (Helderman, 2007) and "layering" (Okma, 2008) of governance modes. In principle, the new scheme widened choice for the insured regarding their health plans, and for patients regarding their health care providers. In practice, Dutch citizens have shown little interest in "shopping around" for health insurance after the first year of the new law's introduction. The small and fairly homogenous country does not allow for much "exit" for any party. Since 1991, Dutch health insurers no longer have to contract with every health care provider. Insurers, however, have shown themselves reluctant to break off long-standing contractual relations and face the angry reactions of their insured. New providers — in contrast to health insurers, where there have been few newcomers to the market — have entered the market offering substitutes for traditional health services, but, thus far, their scale of operation has remained modest.

Public and Private Health Insurance in The Netherlands in the 20th Century

Apart from the system elements and policy goals which Dutch health care shares with other European countries (universal coverage and access to health care, solidarity in sharing the financial burden, cost control, patient choice, and professional autonomy), there are three important characteristics that traditionally have set the system apart: the relatively high share of private funding (at least until 2006; see below), the long tradition of nongovernment provision of care, and the neocorporatist style of social policy-making (Okma, 2001).

The Netherlands shares several institutional features of the funding, contracting, and administration of health care with its neighbor Germany. Both systems are hybrids between the German Bismarck-type employment-related system and the Beveridge model of population-wide health insurance (see the introduction to this volume). Holland's social policy has borrowed heavily from Germany. Since the late 19th century, Holland has looked to the German example of social employment-based health insurance, and successive governments tried to introduce similar legislation. However, they failed to reach agreement about the governance model or, more precisely, about which parties would dominate the boards of the sick funds: labor unions, employers, and government, or only labor and capital. In 1941, the German occupational forces imposed the Sick Fund Decree, which required certain groups of low-income wage earners to register with a sick fund. External imposition of the model (without direct government representation but under tight state control) thus solved the problem.

After the war, the government decided to keep the system in place. By the time it became the base for the formal Sick Fund Law (*Ziekenfondswet*, or ZFW) in 1962, the private insurance market already covered over 30% of the population. The government accepted this reality and made an agreement with the private insurers to keep the share of the public insurance under 65% of the population, informally labeled as the "peace border" (when Germany introduced its social health insurance in 1883, only about 10% of the population had taken out private insurance, and thus its peace border was set at a much lower level than in The Netherlands). For over four decades, until 2006, all changes in policy respected this peace border.

From 1962 to 2006, about two-thirds of the Dutch population had coverage under the mandatory ZFW for acute medical care in hospitals and by general physicians, prescription drugs, and some other services. The sick funds, independent administrative bodies that had run the voluntary mutual income protection schemes since the late 19th century, remained responsible for administering the social insurance. In exchange for taking on this public role, they gained virtually unrestricted access to public funding: when health expenditures rose, their contribution rates (and sometimes government subsidies) went up, too.[3] As those increased contributions translated into higher wage costs, social (health) insurance became one of the core objects of fiscal and social policy.

In 1968, The Netherlands introduced a separate social insurance for long-term care: the Algemene Wet Bijzondere Ziektekosten, or AWBZ (Exceptional Medical Expenses Act). This covers the costs of hospitalization longer than 365 days, stays in mental institutions, and nursing care in special facilities and at home, as well as some other health services. The AWBZ shifted the risks for those costs from families, charities, and local communities to public funding. As a result, there has been a rapid expansion of institutional inpatient care, and today Holland still has one of the highest rates of long-term inpatient care in Europe.

As in other countries, patients pay for some services out of their own pocket or face copayments for other services. But, similar to the other countries in this study, governments have mitigated the effects of such user fees by exempting certain groups or setting limits on how much a family must pay each year.

Although private insurance was voluntary, the rate of noninsurance was less than 2% of the population in the late 1990s (Ministry of Health, 1996). Perhaps this reflects a general tendency of Dutch families to take extensive insurance coverage for illness, their homes, their cars, and other property. In any case, this low rate of noninsurance was an important starting point for the new scheme of 2006 — dramatically different from that in the US, with over 15% of the population uninsured (CDC, 2007).

---

[3] Following OECD publications, this volume labels the income-related payments for social health insurance as "contributions," and flat-rate (nominal) payments for private insurance as "premiums" (OECD, 1992, 1995).

A second important feature of Dutch health care is the dominance of private provision of services.[4] As with other countries in Western Europe, The Netherlands has had a long tradition of provision of collective goods by voluntary, nongovernmental organizations. Their origins can be traced back to medieval guilds offering financial protection to their members in case of illness or death, and local communities, churches, and monasteries setting up hospitals as shelters for the homeless, elderly, sick, and mentally ill (De Swaan, 1988). The majority of Dutch hospitals and other health care institutions were owned and run by charities, nonprofit foundations, or religious orders. The tradition of public services provided by nongovernmental actors is still visible today, even while recent waves of mergers have led to the fading of denominational backgrounds. It is important to note that in spite of the continuing dominance of not-for-profit health care, the system has always contained for-profit elements. For example, the drugs and medical devices industry is almost exclusively for-profit, and most general practitioners and many other health professionals are independent entrepreneurs. The government has a limited role in providing health care; it mostly provides traditional public health and family welfare services via local authorities, and national programs for vaccinations and research.

Third, the arena of social policy in The Netherlands has been characterized by its own tradition of neocorporatist policy-making (Lijphart, 1968; Freddi, 1989; Wildasvky, 1999). In this model, organized stakeholders share the responsibility with governments for the shaping and outcomes of social policy. In health care, for example, the main groups include labor unions, employers, medical associations, other associations of health care providers and insurers, and organized patient groups. In the Dutch tradition, those associations often had a denominational background. The basic assumption of this interaction between state and organized interests was a certain hierarchy in responsibilities, with preference for the lowest possible level (labeled as "sovereignty in its own sphere"

---

[4] Private provision in Europe includes, generally speaking, nongovernment actors, both for-profit and not-for-profit health care facilities. In North America, the term usually refers to investor-owned providers.

by Protestants, or "subsidiarity" by Catholics; the latter term is still common in EU politics, to indicate a preference for national policies over EU-level decision-making). First, individual families had to take care of their own members, and second, the denominational organizations to which Dutch families belonged (such as churches, schools, radio stations, housing corporations, home care associations, or other welfare organizations) were to provide support. Only when those two levels failed to meet the basic needs of the members would the state step in as a residual safety net.

Thus, by the end of the 20th century, Dutch health care combined a mix of public and private funding with nongovernment health care provision, and independent and decentralized administration of health care and health insurance, but under extensive government regulation.

Origins of the Dutch Health Care Reforms: Internal and External Pressure for Change

The decades after World War II saw a gradual expansion of social insurance in The Netherlands, including schemes for disability, unemployment, and sickness benefits, old age pensions, and social health insurance. The majority of the Dutch population welcomed the expanded capacity of hospitals, nursing homes, and other health facilities as an integral part of the modern welfare state. There was some concern about the rising costs of health care, but mostly wide acceptance of the growing role of the state in the funding and planning of health care.

As in other industrialized countries, the oil crises and economic stagnation of the 1970s, combined with changing ideological views on the role of the state and revised demographic projections that revealed a more rapid aging of the population than earlier predicted, created pressure for change and triggered extensive debate about the future of the welfare stare. After decades of typical Dutch consensual neocorporatist policy-making, with major stakeholders sharing the responsibility for social policy with the government (Lijphart, 1968), the focus shifted to models of individualized and decentralized decision-making. In health care, advisory expert groups proposed merging public and private insurance schemes for both acute medical treatment and long-term care, and doing away with the difference between public and private health insurance. This would create a universal insurance, with independent, competing (but not-for-profit), insurers offering a wider range of health plans from which the Dutch insured could choose. The reform process also included adjustments to the policy arena itself, in particular the dismantlement of some of the neocorporatist arrangements. While earlier health reforms were only partially implemented, they helped to change the political climate and opened the way for new forms of for-profit health insurance and health care that did not have much public support in earlier decades.

In 1987, an expert committee headed by the CEO of Philips Electronics, Wisse Dekker, proposed a major overhaul of the health care system (Commissie Dekker, 1987). The committee identified several problems, such as the fragmented funding, a lack of financial incentives to consumers, providers, and health insurers to contain the growth of health expenditures or offer good quality care, and rigid regulations inhibiting a more flexible organization of services. In itself, the Dekker report's analysis was not new: earlier reports had also pointed to those weaknesses, and one common theme in their recommendations was to integrate public and private insurance (Okma, 1997a).

The Dekker committee proposed an amalgamation of existing funding streams into one mandatory (social) health insurance system for the entire population, covering the risks of both acute medical care and long-term care. It sought to strengthen the role of sick funds (and private insurers) as third-party payers in health care, and to increase consumer choice.[5] The proposals included free choice of health insurer, reduction of the services

---

[5] Consumer voice, however, did get short thrift as the dismantling of the advisory bodies also eliminated the direct representation of patient and consumer groups. In the late 1990s, the government initiated so-called "regional patient and consumer platforms" to channel patient interests in health care. As a somewhat odd construction, provincial authorities became responsible for those platforms. Basically, this was a move to appease the provinces after their loss of control over health care planning. Those "patient platforms," however, never really gained much ground in health care decision-making.

covered by the mandatory basic insurance, partial replacement of the income-related contributions by community-rated flat-rate premiums, and options for insured persons to accept deductibles or coinsurance in exchange for lower premiums. Further, the committee wanted to reduce the role of the government by deregulating the existing planning and fee-setting legislation (all but eliminating the role of local and regional authorities in this field).

Basically, the expert group recommended the introduction of an "internal market" within the framework of social health insurance (Schut, 1997; Schut and Van de Ven, 2005). This would not eliminate the role of the state in health care altogether, however, as the government was to determine the coverage of the mandatory health insurance, set the budgets of the health insurers, and monitor health insurance and the quality of health services. The responsibility for negotiations over the quantity, quality, and prices of health services was to shift to (competing) health care providers and (competing, but not-for profit) health insurers, within the framework of social health insurance.[6] The aim was to create a level playing field for sick funds and private insurance. The underlying idea was that consumer choice of health insurer combined with selective

[6] Interestingly, the 1987 Dekker report does not refer to comparative studies of experience abroad. The staff of the expert committee wrote the report, largely based on internal discussions. Afterwards, some claimed that Alain Enthoven's "Consumer Choice Plan" of the 1970s served as its example (Van de Ven and Schut, 2008). But there is no evidence of such parentage. There is in fact another, more likely explanation for similarities between reform proposals in different countries, namely the limited number of options available for any country seeking to combine universal access with efficient management. On the funding side, (earmarked) general taxation and mandated contributions for social health insurance fulfill the requirement of income-related payments that can safeguard universal coverage. On the contracting side, there are three models: the integrated model of the British NHS, the reimbursement model of private insurance, and long term contractual relations between third party payers and providers (OECD, 1992, 1994). Therefore, the search for models that combine universal access to health care with a fair distribution of the financial burden and increased efficiency of health care will come up with a limited number of models. The dominant experience in OECD member states in the 1980s and 1990s was the shift towards the "public contracting model," with public funding and independent health care providers.

contracting would create incentives to improve the quality and efficiency of services as well as contain health expenditures.

At first, the proposals caused much uproar in the world of Dutch health care (Okma, 1997a). It also drew much interest from abroad. After lengthy debate, Parliament accepted the proposals. The Ministry of Health framed an ambitious four-year implementation plan for 1989–1992 (Ministry of Health, 1988). In the end, however, it realized only a few (but important) steps. For example, in 1991, it shifted ambulatory mental health care, prescription drugs, and some other services from the public and private health insurance systems to the long-term care insurance, which was to become the new social health insurance for all.[7] Further, the government relaxed the rules for hospital planning and setting fees. Local authorities lost control over the establishment of new practices for family doctors, and fee ceilings replaced fixed fees for health services. Provincial authorities lost their role in the planning of hospitals and other health facilities. In a later stage, to "compensate" for this loss, provinces were given the task of organizing regional platforms of consumer and patient groups. Other steps included the abolition of legal boundaries of the working areas of sick funds (so that they could expand their activities country-wide) and the introduction of selective contracting of self-employed health professionals by the funds (with the announcement that the mandatory contracting of health facilities would later end). These measures increased the room for insurers to negotiate with providers over the volume, price, and quality of services, and to selectively contract with providers.

After the first steps of implementing the reforms in the early 1990s, stakeholder opposition resurfaced, public support eroded, and the political backing became more and more hesitant (Okma, 1997a). After accepting (albeit in adjusted form) the legislation for the second reform phase in 1991, Parliament decided to shelve discussion of the next steps. Following

[7] At the time, this approach seemed a sensible choice as the AWBZ already applied to the entire population, and a gradual shift of entitlements from other public and private health insurance schemes to the AWBZ would require the least degree of legislative and administrative change.

the general elections in 1994, a new, surprising governing coalition consisting of the Labor Party (PvdA), Conservatives (VVD), and Liberal Democrats (D66) stepped into office. For the first time in over half a century, the Christian Democrat Party (CDA) was not in power. The governing manifesto of this new "Purple Coalition" stated that it would no longer continue the reforms, but shift towards incremental adjustment of the existing system instead (Regeerakkoord, 1994). Four years later, the same coalition continued in office and maintained its policy course (Regeerakkoord, 1998). This time, however, it also announced that it would study the need for structural reform. It framed its intention to introduce a universal basic health insurance in the policy paper *Vraag aan Bod* ("Demand at the Center") (Ministry of Health, 2001).

In December 2001, the Purple Coalition stepped down from office over the political fallout of the tragic events in Srebrenica, where a small and insufficiently armed battalion of Dutch soldiers were not able to defend the village's population and the Serbian attackers murdered all the 5000 or so male Muslim inhabitants. The general elections of May 2002 brought sweeping gains for a new party, List Pim Fortuyn (LPF), only a few weeks after the murder of its populist leader, Pim Fortuyn. This surprising election outcome brought the Christian Democrats back to power, together with VVD and LPF. The new CDA–VVD–LPF coalition presented its governing manifesto in June 2002 (*Strategisch Akkoord*, 2002). But escalating internal conflicts led to its rapid demise. After the January 2003 elections, in spite of a large electoral gain by the Labor Party, the CDA and VVD switched partners, replacing List Pim Fortuyn with the Liberal Democrats. This, in fact, recreated the dominant CDA–VVD–D66 coalition of the early 1980s. The new coalition presented its plans in a May 2003 governing manifesto, *Meedoen, Meer Werk, Minder Regels* ("Participation, More Work, Less Rules") (*Hoofdlijnenakkoord*, 2003). In health policy, the program included a striking mix of old and new instruments to control costs and improve efficiency: delisting of services, new or increased copayments and deductibles, strict budgetary ceilings, and, again, the intention to introduce universal health insurance based on the principle of "regulated market competition" (without defining or explaining that term in more detail). In 2007, Labor

Table 1.   Dutch Health Care Reforms of the 1980s and 1990s

Years	Governing Coalition	Health Reform Steps
1987–1989	CDA–VVD (deputy minister Dick Dees)	1987: Dekker Report proposals: population-wide social health insurance, including long-term care
1989–1994	CDA and PvdA (deputy minister Hans Simons)	1991: First steps of implementation (abandoning regional borders of sick fund and local planning of general practitioners' offices)
1994–1998	First Purple Coalition: VVD, PvdA, and D66 (minister Els Borst-Eilers)	Formal abandonment of Dekker reforms; shift to incremental policy (but continuation of some reform steps)
1998–2001	Second Purple Coalition: VVD, PvdA, and D66 (minister Els Borst-Eilers)	Continuation of incremental policy; announcement of feasibility study on universal health insurance
2001	Fall of Purple Coalition	
2002	CDA, VVD, and LPF coalition (minister Eduard Bomhoff)	Proposals for universal health insurance (excluding AWBZ) allowing for-profit insurers
2003	CDA, VVD, and D66 (minister Hans Hoogervorst)	Continued preparation of universal (private) insurance
2004	CDA, VVD, and D66 (minister Hans Hoogervorst)	Second Chamber of Parliament passes Health Insurance Law (universal mandate to take out health insurance), administered by former sick funds and private health insurers
2005	CDA, VVD, and D66 (minister Hans Hoogervorst)	First Chamber of Parliament passes Health Insurance Law
2006	CDA, VVD, and D66 (minister Hans Hoogervorst)	1 January 2006: Health Insurance Law comes into effect
2007	CDA and PvdA (minister Ab Klink)	Continued implementation of health insurance; moratorium on changes in AWBZ

Source: Authors.

again replaced the Conservatives in the coalition with the Christian Democrats; this time, the two parties opted for the small conservative Christian party (CU) as their coalition partner.

One particular factor played a crucial role in the rapid passage of the 2006 health insurance. In the late 1990s, there was rising dissatisfaction with growing waiting lists in Dutch health care, especially the care of elderly and chronically ill patients. To solve this problem, the Cabinet decided to drastically increase the funding for health care. As a result, waiting lists went down, and public spending on health care went up considerably. A few years later, however, politicians seemed to have forgotten the former episode, focusing on the "runaway growth" of public health expenditures (caused, in fact, by explicit policy decisions to increase funding rather than uncontrollable cost pressures). The new health minister, Hans Hoogervorst (who had been deputy minister of finance before becoming minister of health in 2003), used the cost escalation as his main argument in favor of the new ("private") health insurance system and succeeded in convincing Parliament to pass the law in 2005. In this way, he helped create a "window of opportunity" for policy change (Kingdon, 1984). There seemed to be a general "sense of urgency" (perhaps more in the political world than amongst the Dutch population in general) and there was seemingly widespread agreement over the available solutions. The Christian Democrats, who had just returned to power, were more than willing to act, while the dismantlement of the neo-corporatist institutions had reduced the veto power of organized interests. The minister himself also proved to be a skillful "policy entrepreneur."

Substantially, the 2006 law is very similar to the earlier Dekker reform proposals which failed largely because of resurfacing stakeholder opposition, but it pushed the notion of market competition even further (Okma, 1997a). In 2005, when the new law passed Parliament, there was remarkably little public debate or opposition to the proposals. The Senate (or the First Chamber of Parliament) basically passed the bill in one day — the day before summer recess — a stunningly short time for passing such far-reaching change in social health insurance.

Thus, the changes in political coalitions and the shift from structural reform to incremental policies did not defeat the core elements of the

law and somewhat more than an informal agreement, covenants are not legally binding, but the government sees them as a convenient way to engage and involve major stakeholders in realizing its goals. For example, when expenditures for hospitals exceeded the budget estimates in 2004, the Ministry of Health framed a covenant with the hospital association and national association of health insurers (Ministry of Health, 2006). There are similar covenants with pharmacists and the pharmaceutical industry that aim to restrain the growth of pharmaceutical expenditure.

While the rules of the game in social policies changed, the new rules did not replace the old ones. In the early 2000s, illustrating a certain degree of internal inconsistency in policy-making (perhaps reflecting a somewhat weak belief in the cost-controlling capacities of market competition in health care), the Dutch government turned its attention, once again, to a reassessment of the benefit package of social health insurance, tight budget controls, delisting services and introducing or increasing user fees (Scheerder, 2005).

As noted above, the creation of the internal market in Dutch health care did not lead to a reduced presence of the government. On the contrary, there is wide recognition that competitive markets require extensive regulation and supervision to function fairly well. In spite of announced shifts from "supply regulation" to "demand regulation," both categories of government regulation are now firmly in place.[14] Dutch citizens — like other Europeans — expect the government to safeguard access to good quality health care and to step in if needed. For example, faced with public discontent over the delisting of dental checkups for adults or IVF treatments from the basic insurance, the government rapidly decided to reinstate (part of) those services (Maarse and Okma, 2005). In close collaboration with private interests, the government also extended its presence in monitoring health care quality, the development of case-based payment models, and the implementation of information technology.

---

[14] Those terms are not self-explanatory. "Supply regulation" refers to government control of the allocation of resources, planning of health facilities, and setting of prices (as well as quality supervision). "Demand regulation" is based on the assumption that individual choice of health plans and providers will lead to an efficient allocation of resources as (competing) health insurers contract (competing) providers on behalf of their insured.

The government thus encouraged providers and insurers to compete but, at the same time, kept tight control over health expenditure and the allocation of public funds. This has resulted in complementing administrative models (Helderman, 2007) or, perhaps more accurately, in a complicated *overlay* of governance modes based on quite divergent and sometimes conflicting notions of the role of the state and citizens. This overlay has created managerial dilemmas for Dutch health care providers and insurers. For example, they have to invest in improving services and expanding market shares, but they also face growing uncertainty over future clients and income streams. They have to act as entrepreneurs, but they also have to sit down with public authorities at the national, regional, and local levels to discuss policy results. They compete, but governments also want them to collaborate with their colleagues in the region and to participate in collective decision-making. They have to attract and keep their patients and insured, but they also have to please the government and other stakeholders.

Changing Stakeholder Positions in Dutch Health Policy

The Dutch health reform legislation of the 1980s and 1990s introduced entrepreneurial risks to players who had previously enjoyed high levels of certainty and income protection. The population groups eligible for the social insurance were automatically insured; their employers paid their contributions as earmarked taxes, less "visible" than the nominal (flat rate) premiums for private insurance. The sick fund members had virtually unrestricted access to health care, with modest amounts of user fees for certain services. Since 1991, sick fund insured can change plans; the 2006 reforms added the option to take up higher deductible plans in exchange for lower premiums. The sick funds, in turn, had almost unrestricted access to public funding; they also had to contract with all health care providers, who in turn were certain to receive their annual budget. From 1991 to 2006 (when the budget system expanded to the other insurers), sick funds received a capitated budget that took into account certain risk factors, like age, gender, employment status, and health status of their insured (Leu *et al.*, 2008; Schut and Van de Ven, 2005). That budget replaced the open-ended reimbursement that characterized the former sick fund model of the early 20th century. In 2006, this part covered about 50% of expenditures. In a way, the new budget model heralded the restoration of the status of sick funds as independent risk-bearing insurers (Okma and Van der Burg, 2004). It has broken up the wider pool of social insurance by shifting insurance risk (back) to the individual health insurers.

Dutch health insurers have addressed those challenges in different ways. They sought to gain strategic market positions by improving their administration, merging with others, and improving and expanding (and sometimes contracting) their coverage and services. In general, insurers have shown themselves more concerned with defending and expanding their market shares than with improving the quality and efficiency of health care. In the years before and after the introduction of the new population-wide health insurance, insurers spent massive amounts on marketing and advertising. Several set their premiums below cost and many insurers are still in the red. Nevertheless, on average, premiums rose by about 10% in 2007 and experts expect a further premium hike (Smit and Mokveld, 2007).

Some health insurers tried to reduce waiting lists and waiting times by pressuring hospitals to work more efficiently and contracting with for-profit clinics. Others offered new services, like 24-hour call centers for their insured. A few experimented with preferred provider arrangements, though this never became very popular with Dutch patients. With pre-ferred provider arrangements, insured face higher charges when they go to a provider outside the contracted network of their health insurance. Some insurers widened their supplemental coverage by including a variety of preventive services, such as sports clinics or regular checkups. As the latest step, insurers have explored forms of integration with health services. This, in effect, has led to the creation of institutions that resemble the health maintenance organization (HMO) model which started in the U.S. in the 1970s (even while the actual expansion of such activities is still modest in The Netherlands).[15] In a broader historical perspective,

[15] See also the introduction to this volume about the diverging notions of the term "health maintenance organization."

however, such HMOs are very similar to the original, 19th century sick funds that combined income protection arrangements for their members with the ownership of health facilities and employment of physicians.

Most if not all health insurers focused on the market for collective insurance contracts to keep their clients and attract new ones. Almost 60% of those who changed their health insurance in 2006 did so as members of collective employment-based plans (Smit and Mokveld, 2007). In 2007, this share had risen to over 80% while less than 5% of the Dutch insured were switching — thus, less than 1% of the population decided to switch plans as an individual decision. Clearly, there has been a trend towards increased collectivization of health insurance, in a way strengthening and not weakening the employment base of health insurance in The Netherlands.

In principle, the abolition of the regional monopolies of sick funds in 1991 allowed new entrants into the social health insurance field. In practice, however, it accelerated the process of mergers and acquisitions that sharply reduced competition. At the beginning of the 20th century there were over 1200 independent sick funds in The Netherlands. That number went down from 600 in 1950, to about 60 in the early 1980s and 30 in 1999 (Okma, 2001). In the late 1990s, the funds averaged 300,000 members, but membership ranged from a few thousands to over one million insured. In 1999, there were also about 40 private insurers that catered to the remaining 40% of the population. In 2005, after a rapid process of mergers and informal collaboration between public and private insurance, there were 43 health insurers (both former sick funds and private insurers). Many of those operated as part of conglomerates. For example, five main health insurance groups (Achmea, VGZ-IZA, CA, Menzis, and Agis) covered 11 million insured, or over 60% of the population in that year (Rengers and Van Uffelen, 2005). After further consolidations, there were 15 health insurers in The Netherlands, and the two largest conglomerates (VGZ-IZA and Agis-Menza) covered over 50% of the population.

International insurance conglomerates that offer both public and private health insurance in the European Union have also explored the Dutch market. But some of the foreign firms that tried their hand at offering health insurance in Holland in the 1990s, such as the French AXA and the German DKV, soon left the country again.

Uninsured in The Netherlands

The occurrence of uninsured persons has always been a sensitive policy issue in The Netherlands. Traditionally, this number has been very low. Although the 40% of the population who were not eligible for social insurance did not have to take out (private) insurance until 2006, the vast majority had actually done so. Only about 1% of the Dutch population was uninsured. While the new health insurance is mandatory, there are few effective sanctions if a person does not take out insurance. At first, the Health Ministry decided that in case someone without insurance needed hospitalization, he or she would not only have to pay the hospital costs himself or herself, but also take out insurance on the spot, retroactively, and pay a fine. But that solution did not appear feasible as most politicians realized that enforcing additional fees on low-income families would be hard to do. Under the new system, private health insurers can bar someone who has not paid their monthly premium for over three months. In 2007, the chairman of the national association of Dutch health insurers (*Zorgverzekeraars Nederland*, or ZN) announced that its members intended to stop covering persons who had not paid their premiums. To prevent this from happening, the government first considered the creation of a separate risk pool for the uninsured (Ministry of Health, 2006). It eventually talked the insurers into keeping those delinquents on their rolls. The government also commissioned a study of the composition of the delinquent population from the Central Bureau of Statistics (CBS) (CBS, 2007). The CBS compared the number of people registered with a local authority to the number enrolled with a health insurer to find the number of uninsured. In mid-2007, there were about 200,000 people who had not paid their premium for over six months (and thus absent government action would become uninsured). Added to the 240,000 or so uninsured in the country, this would almost have doubled the number of uninsured. Though still a modest share, it nonetheless became a significant issue in Dutch social policy (a very similar experience to that of Israel; see the chapter in this volume). Next, the CBS looked at the data provided by the insurers in more detail. Predictably, the study revealed overrepresentation of young immigrants, single-parent families, and welfare recipients. It was clear that a large share of those low-income families would not be able to pay large amounts of fines, premiums, or hospital costs out of pocket. In a letter to Parliament in 2007, the Minister of Health therefore proposed returning to a system where welfare recipients would no longer have to pay the flat-rate premium themselves (Ministry of Health, 2007a). Local welfare offices would deduct the monthly amount from the welfare income (a solution that the cities of Rotterdam and Amsterdam had already proposed in 2005). In another letter to Parliament, the Minister announced that the insurers would keep the delinquents insured but the government would try to recover the due premiums (Ministry of Health, 2007a, 2007b). Moreover, delinquents would not be allowed to leave their insurer before paying all the outstanding amounts.

Changing Attitudes of Health Care Managers

Managers of hospitals and other health care services — like health insurers — have reacted in different ways to the new challenges (De Roo, 2002, 1993). They contracted out maintenance and hotel functions and developed arrangements for collective purchase of medical goods. Managers built up financial reserves by improving their administration and expanding office hours, realizing economies of scale. They reined in labor costs by differentiating functions and replacing skilled staff with less expensive labor. Some hospitals have created for-profit subsidiaries. Others shifted from standardized to customized care, added luxury care, and extended services to become more attractive to patients and health insurers alike. A few providers ventured into new areas of health-care-related services, including home care, meals on wheels, and sports clinics.

Like the insurers, providers tried to focus on the most promising market segments by selecting the wealthiest, healthiest, and cheapest groups, and by setting up health clinics to provide rapid access for employees. Public polls and debates in the Dutch Parliament revealed strong opposition to such queue jumping or services limited to certain groups. In the late 1990s, the Health Minister announced measures to limit the activities of private clinics and to prohibit preferential treatment altogether. A few years later, however, that opposition seemed to have faded. In fact, later governments considered the rise of private clinics (independent treatment centers, *zelfstandige behandelcentra*, or ZBCs) as a solution to the problem of long waiting lists, because they added to the total treatment capacity. But not all of those centers fared well, and after a few years some closed their doors.

Further, Dutch health care providers — like insurers — strengthened their market position by collaborating or even fully merging with other providers. Many hospitals and other health facilities developed informal networks and engaged in horizontal integration with similar institutions and vertical integration with nursing homes, retirement facilities, and extramural care in their region.[16] In fact, in several cases, such regional collaboration has sharply reduced the number of independent providers, sometimes eliminating competition altogether and thereby also reducing consumer choice. In particular, providers of care for the elderly and the mentally ill have shown themselves eager entrepreneurs. In some instances, their activities led to virtual regional monopolies, defeating procompetitive government policies. In the field of hospital care, this has created a tension between the contracting role of health insurers (based on the assumption that they negotiate with competing providers over contracts) and efforts of the Health Ministry to encourage regional collaboration between health care service providers (Boot, 1998).

---

[16] Interestingly, this form of vertical integration of hospital care with nursing home and home care occurred in anticipation of the basic health insurance (based on the Dekker proposals) that was to provide coverage for both acute medical care and long-term nursing care. It is not yet clear whether providers have to legally "undo" such integrated services after the decision to keep the long-term care insurance, AWBZ, separate. In 2004, the government decided to shift responsibility for those entitlements to local authorities, but in 2007 it announced a moratorium on further change in the long-term care insurance.

In spite of the aforementioned "market-oriented" activities, the associations of providers and health insurers have maintained their prominent presence in the health care arena. They have continued to engage in a wide range of collaborative efforts; despite the growing market rhetoric, they have continued to work with the government to find a common solution to problems of cost control, the rising number of uninsured, and other issues. In a political sense, there clearly has not been a major "exit" (Hirschman, 1970). One of the reasons is that there are not that many exit options from the policy arena in a small country where the leaders of all the main stakeholder groups know each other well and continue to meet regularly.

New Roles for Patients and Consumers in Dutch Health Care

Dutch citizens and patients have taken new roles, too, but this has hardly resulted in "consumer-driven" health care. Since the abolition of regional boundaries of sick funds in 1991, almost all of the 30 or so funds expanded their activities countrywide, so that people with social insurance could switch plans.[17] To encourage this mobility, the government sponsored websites offering comparative information about health care and health insurance. In the early 1990s, the main consumer association in The Netherlands, *Consumentenbond*, started to publish systematic assessments of the costs and quality of health care and health insurance. The weekly *Elsevier* published lists of the "best and worst" hospitals. The national daily *Algemeen Dagblad* gained fame by publishing detailed lists of waiting times for certain medical procedures, encouraging patients to actively shop around when faced with unacceptable waiting lists. Nonetheless, this rapid growth in comparative information has had a

---

[17] A seemingly contradictory consequence of the extended option to switch sick funds was that persons with social insurance now had more choice than private insured who — as in the US — face barriers or denial of coverage altogether due to pre-existing medical conditions or for other reasons. In the private market, this can cause the problem of "job lock" when people cannot change work for fear of losing their health insurance.

limited effect on patient behavior. Dutch citizens seem rather weary of the bombardment of new information, suggesting a backlash against the rise of consumerism in Dutch health care (Okma and Ooijens, 2005).

Until the early 2000s, mobility of insured persons remained very modest (Laske-Aldershof *et al.*, 2004). That changed dramatically with the introduction of the basic health insurance of 2006 — at least for the first year. Almost 20% of insured changed their health insurance in 2006. Over half of those did so as members of collective employment-based plans (Smit and Mokveld, 2007). In 2007, less than 5% of the Dutch insured changed plans (of those who did, over 80% acted as part of employment-related collective contracts). Thus, interestingly, the new insurance has strengthened rather than weakened the collective nature of Dutch health insurance even while its basic premise is that of individual choice as the driving force to improve the quality and efficiency of health care. The collective insurance contracts now also include groups of patients with a particular disease or other special groups — a new phenomenon in Dutch health care. Some insurers even offered a "collective" contract for insured without access to another group. Insurers do not have to accept every group seeking coverage, however, and some patient groups have been turned down. For example, insurers are clearly less interested in chronically ill patients (Bartolomee and Maarse, 2007). The large-scale change of insurer thus seems to have been a one-shot event in 2006, mostly as part of collective employment-based arrangements rather than being based on individual choice.

In general, people who are part of employment-based collective groups represent lower risks and are more attractive to insurance companies. There clearly is an element of risk selection by health insurers and self-selection by insured in this pattern of collective contracting. But, thus far, this has not created major problems (though it is still a bit early to assess the final outcome of this process). Dutch health insurers traditionally have felt the bounds of social norms that condemn such behavior, and in the past they never applied risk rating that fully reflected the risk of certain groups (Okma, 1997a). The growth of collective contracting has pushed up the premiums for individual coverage. To counteract this trend — as another example of government intervention in the private market — the government has ruled that health insurers cannot offer more than a 10% discount on collective contracts (Smit and Mokveld, 2007).

Dutch patients show a high degree of loyalty to hospitals (particularly hospitals with a religious background) and to their former regional sick funds (Laske-Aldershof *et al.*, 2004). Perhaps this confirms March and Simon's (1958) assumption of "satisficing behavior": most people limit their choice to the first few alternatives they can clearly comprehend. They simply refuse to go much beyond the first option that seems reasonable (or that they already know well), and they do not have the time to shop around extensively. The bombardment of information provided by government-sponsored or commercial websites, newspapers, specialized journals, or other media has not done much to change satisficing behavior in Dutch health care.

Interestingly, the area where consumer action has affected services the most is not acute medical care, but long-term care (Okma, 1997b). In this domain, organized patient groups have successfully lobbied for better quality of services, in particular the "lunatics movement" of psychiatric patients in the 1960s, and relatives of developmentally handicapped patients. The strategy of "voice" (Hirschman, 1970) has worked well in this area. In other areas of long-term care, there has been some "exit" as well. Since the mid-1990s, the long-term care insurance, AWBZ, has offered the option for certain categories of patients to take cash benefits or vouchers instead of services in kind. This allows them to contract with providers outside the traditional institutions. Within a few years, those vouchers became very popular. By the end of 2003, over 50,000 patients had taken this option, receiving an average amount of over €20,000 (US$28,000) per year. In 2006, the total budget for those vouchers was over €1 billion (US$1.4 billion), or about half the entire budget for home care — while home care organizations provided care to over 600,000 persons (Ministry of Health, 2006). Thus, voice and exit became two effective strategies in long-term care. In acute medical care, however, loyalty dominates as Dutch patients express far less interest in exiting the care they are familiar with. Interestingly, government policy mostly focuses on increasing competition in acute care. It seems less convinced of the market power of consumers in long-term care. In 2007, the government announced a moratorium on changes in AWBZ, and it will keep long-term care under strict government control (Ministry of Health, 2007).

Conclusions and the Outlook for the Dutch Health Care System

At the beginning of the 21st century, the main actors in the Dutch health policy arena — insurers and providers — have shown a mix of anticipatory and defensive behavior. They anticipated shifts from centralized consensual policy-making with strong government control to decentralized decision-making and the creation of internal markets. This anticipatory behavior explains much of the smooth transition to the new health insurance system of 2006. Because of this anticipatory behavior, the notions of individualized choice that did not gain lasting support during the earlier reform efforts became more acceptable in the mid-2000s. Rather than heralding a new era of competition, however, the new system codified behavior that already was in place. The same type of law that in the late 1980s would have been considered an instrument of "modification" had become an instrument of "codification," not because it had changed direction itself, but because the context and behavior of the group affected by the law had changed (see Okma, 1997a, Chap. 7 for this argument).

A second question this chapter seeks to address is whether the 2006 system implies a dramatic change in Dutch health care. "Yes and no" is the short answer. Yes because the 2006 legislation effectively ended the more than 100-year-old tradition of sick funds, plunging Dutch health care into uncharted territory. This has prompted health insurers and health care providers to anticipate and to adjust. Some have improved and expanded the range of their services and some have limited their services — particularly in the areas of mental care and care of the elderly. Most have sought to consolidate their market positions by mergers and acquisitions. Insurers merged mostly at the national level, while providers sought to limit competition by creating new strategic alliances on the regional level, in several cases eliminating competition altogether. One cannot yet say whether and to what extent these activities have improved the quality, efficiency, and patient-friendliness of Dutch health care services (Okma and Ooijens, 2005). The main actors seem to be focused more on gaining and defending strategic market positions than on increasing consumer choice and improving the quality and efficiency of health care. But another way of looking at the legislation is to trace its history back to earlier reform efforts of the 1980s and 1990s.

The strategic behavior of health insurers and health care providers — anticipating changes in government policy — has contributed to the reshaping of the health policy arena. This has also created new problems. For example, the announced amalgamation of the acute care and long-term care insurance systems in the original Dekker proposals encouraged hospital managers to seek vertical integration by merging with outpatient care and nursing home services. In 2006, the government reversed its plan. It left the long-term care insurance, AWBZ, out of the basic insurance, announcing that local authorities instead of health insurers would have a greater say in this field (but it again changed its position in 2007). Thus, the integrated providers now face another split in their revenues and have to deal with different negotiating partners. Such turnarounds in policy, not uncommon in Dutch social policy, have made managers of health insurance and health care wary of major shifts in their business. They try new directions but cannot afford to break off existing long-term relations. There is thus much continuity and only gradual change.

Moreover, the creation of an internal market in Dutch health care has not led to a reduced presence of the government. In spite of an announced shift from supply regulation to demand regulation, both categories of government regulation are firmly in place. Dutch citizens expect a strong government role in safeguarding access to good quality care and want the government to step in if needed. For example, faced with rising numbers of uninsured in 2006, the government announced that it was considering the creation of a separate risk pool for uninsured. In 2007, it took up the earlier suggestion of local authorities to abolish the direct payment of flat-rate premiums by welfare recipients altogether to avoid the problem of delinquency (by withholding those amounts from the welfare incomes). The government has also extended its presence in monitoring health care quality, developing case-based payment, and implementing information technology. Thus, markets have not quite replaced the role of the government in Dutch health care.

Another factor explaining the high degree of continuity in Dutch health politics is the permanent presence of multiparty coalitions that impose restraints on changes in social policy (Helderman, 2007). Since the early 20th century, none of the main political parties has ever been large enough to govern by itself. There is always a need for a coalition with others, and changes in political coalition do not appear to have much direct impact on health policy. For example, after the presentation of the Dekker reform plans by the Christian Democratic–Conservative coalition in 1987, the next coalition of the Christian Democrats and the Labor Party actually started to implement the plans in 1989 with only marginal change (for example, leaving long-term care insurance for a later stage). The surprising 1994 coalition, which excluded the Christian Democrats, formally abandoned the reform but did not undo steps already taken; actually, it continued most of its predecessor's policies by relabeling structural reform as incremental adjustments. When the Christian Democratic Party returned to power, it more or less took up the reform course it had started decades before. The comeback of the Labor Party as coalition partner in 2007 did not stop or reverse the introduction of the universal health insurance in 2006 (Regeerakkoord, 2007).

Third, interestingly, the Dutch experience shows that rather than eliminating the role of employers, the reform has actually strengthened their role, as most now offer health insurance as part of a wider package of employee benefits. In both Switzerland and The Netherlands, the new "private" systems under strict government control have greatly added to administrative complexity and costs. The first year after the introduction of the new system in The Netherlands, premiums went up on average by about 10% — not quite the picture of successful cost control by private markets.

It is also important to note that the (partially implemented) health reforms of the 1980s and 1990s did not replace the existing policy directions or governance models in The Netherlands. This has led to a certain degree of "complementarity" of governance models (Helderman, 2007). But it might be more accurate to say that the current landscape of Dutch health care and health insurance reveals a complicated mix of competing and sometimes conflicting notions of public and private governance. The partially implemented and sometimes reversed reform measures have led to an intricate overlay of state control and deregulation, of patient choice and paternalistic government, of market competition and market concentration, of individual choice and collective action, and of a rapid growth of collective, employment-based health insurance arrangements within a system of universal insurance that seeks to enlarge individual choice.

As to the future, it remains to be seen whether the egalitarian tradition in Dutch social policies will create barriers to further shifts towards private for-profit health care. Thus far the experience has shown that there is little support in Dutch society for greater differentiation in treatment or inequalities in access to health care. As we have seen above, Dutch citizens have not shown much interest in switching their health insurance individually after the first year of the new health insurance.

The health policy discourse has shifted (for an elaboration of this point, see Pickard *et al.*, 2006), but the new orientation towards market competition has clearly not replaced former notions of social solidarity in Dutch society. For-profit health services will only be successful on a modest scale as long as the basic insurance covers a wide range of services. Efforts to engage in risk selection on a large scale by insurers and providers will likely face strong resistance and provoke government action. It is not yet clear whether this will change with the growing presence of international insurance conglomerates, in particular when those businesses do not share the traditional business norms in Holland. There is consumerism at the margin, but there is no sign of widespread acceptance of rising inequality in access to health care, and there is no evidence that Dutch citizens are embracing consumer-driven health care. But they have strong feelings about the quality of long-term care for their elderly and handicapped relatives and are willing to take an active position (as seen by the rapid growth of the cash benefit system).

The trend towards greater market concentration in health insurance and health care that accelerated in the 1990s has not yet leveled off. The virtual elimination of competition will probably drive up costs. It will undermine the effectiveness of both market competition and the informal agreements between the government and other parties, as dominant players in a particular market have less need to agree with the government or others.

The Dutch experience illustrates that health policy-making takes place within the constraints of national traditions, national culture, and national institutions.[18] Government policy interacts with the behavior of the groups affected by that policy. This also means that formally stated policies can differ substantially from actual developments. In several cases, even after passing a formal law, the Dutch government changed actual implementation for a variety of reasons. This confirms the importance of clearly distinguishing announced policy proposals from actually implemented ones. Terms like "policy," "health care reform" or "consumer-driven health care" are usually not very well defined.[19] This chapter has shown how announced reforms (even while only partially implemented) and anticipatory behavior by health providers and insurers alike have reshaped the Dutch health care landscape and opened the way for new directions in government policy.[20] Policy proposals that were unacceptable at one time gained support in a later period as some of the main stakeholders had changed their positions and showed anticipatory behavior. Still, new developments are tested against strong popular support for universal access to health care without undue barriers, as well

[18] One particular institutional factor this chapter has not addressed extensively is the growing influence of European Union law on the social policy of EU member states (see also footnote 7).

[19] The term "policy" can mean a general statement of interests and objectives, a set of past actions of the government, a specific statement of future intentions, or a set of standing rules (Palmer and Short, 1989). Many policy studies (or journalistic reports) ignore the fundamental difference between these meanings and simply take policy as the policy outcome.

[20] Rudolf Klein observed that "incremental change" means two quite different things: one, a step-by-step adjustment in a specific direction that, in the end, can result in substantial change or reform; and two, step-by-step change in random directions (Klein, 1995).

by a strong sense of justice and equality in Dutch society. Both public and private actors feel the restraint of such cultural factors and are quick to assure the Dutch population that innovation will not lead to the erosion of social solidarity. When facing public outcry over developments that are generally seen as unfair, the government is quick to act and impose restrictions or reverse its policies.

References

Bartolomee Y, Maarse H. (2007). "Health Insurance Reform in the Netherlands." *Eurohealth* **12**(2) 7–9.

Boot JM. (1998). "Schaalvergroting en Concentratie in het Nederlandse Ziekenhuiswezen" ["Concentration and Increase in Operational Scale of Dutch Hospitals"]. *Bestuurskunde* **7**(1): 28–37.

CBS. (2007). *Kenmerken van Wanbetalers Zorgverzekeringswet* ["Characteristics of the Non-payers of Health Insurance"]. Centraal Bureau voor de Statistiek, Voorburg.

CDC. (2007). "Percentage of Persons of All Ages Without Health Insurance Coverage at the Time of Interview: United States, 1997–June 2007." National Health Interview Survey. Accessed 26 December 2008. www.cdc.gov/nchs/data/nhis/earlyrelease/200712_01.pdf

Commissie De Jong. (1993). "Raad op Maat" ["Measured Advice"]. *Rapport van de Bijzondere Commissie Vraagpunten Adviesorganen.* The Hague: SDU.

Commissie Dekker. (1987). *Bereidheid tot Verandering* ["Willingness to Change; Report of the Committee on Health Care Reform"]. The Hague: Distributiecentrum Overheidspublicaties.

De Roo AA. (1993). "De Zorgsector als Bedrijfstak in Wording" ["Health Care as Emerging Market Branch"]. Lecture. Catholic University Brabant, Tilburg.

De Roo AA. (1995). "Contracting and Solidarity: Market-Oriented Changes in Dutch Health Insurance Systems." In: Saltman RB, Von Otter C. (eds.), *Implementing Planned Markets in Health Care.* Open University Press, Buckingham.

De Roo AA. (2002). "Naar een Nieuw Zorgstelsel?" ["Towards a New Health Care System?"]. Lecture. Tilburg University, Tilburg.

De Swaan A. (1998). *In Care of the State: Health Care, Education and Welfare in Europe and the USA in the Modern Era.* Polity, Oxford.

Enthoven A, Van de Ven WPMM. (2007). "Going Dutch — Managed-Competition Health Insurance in the Netherlands." *NEJM* **357**(24): 2421–2426.

Freddi G. (1989). "Problems of Organizational Rationality in Health Systems: Political Controls and Policy Options." In: Freddi G, Bjorkman J (eds.), *Controlling Medical Professionals: The Comparative Politics of Health Governance.* Sage, London.

Grit C, Dolfsma W. (2002). "The Dynamics of the Dutch Health Care System — A Discourse Analysis." *Rev Soc Econ* **LX**(3): 377–400.

Harris G. (2007). "Looking at Dutch and Swiss Health Systems." *The New York Times*, 30 October.

Helderman J-K. (2007). "Institutional Complementarity in Dutch Health Care Reforms: Going Beyond the Pre-occupation with Choice." European Health Policy Group, Berlin.

Helderman J-K, Schut FT, Van der Grinten TED, Van de Ven WPMM. (2005). "Market-Oriented Health Care Reforms and Policy Learning in the Netherlands." *J Health Polit Policy Law* **30**(1–2): 189–210.

Hirschman AO. (1970). *Exit, Voice and Loyalty: Responses to Decline in Firms, Organizations, and States.* Harvard University Press, Cambridge.

Hoofdlijnenakkoord 2003 ["Governing Manifesto 2003"]. (2003). SDU, The Hague.

Kingdon J. (1984). *Agendas, Alternatives, and Public Policies.* Longman, New York.

Klee M, Okma KGH. (2001). "Covenanten: Nieuw Instrument Van Beleid?" ["Covenante: A New Policy Instrument?"]. *Zorg en Verzekering* **8**(1): 8–20.

Klein R. (1995). *Learning From Others: Shall the Last Be the First Markets?* Four-Country Conference on Health Care Policies and Health Care Reforms in the United States, Canada, Germany and The Netherlands.

Amsterdam, 23–25 February. Ministry of Health, Welfare and Sport, The Hague.

Laske-Aldershof T, Schut E, Beck K, Shmueli A, Van de Voorde C. (2004). "Consumer Mobility in Social Health Insurance Markets: A Five-Country Comparison." *Appl Health Econ Health Policy* **3**(4): 229–241.

Leu RE, Rutten FH, Brouwer W, Matter P, Ruetschi C. (2009). *The Swiss and Dutch Health Insurance Systems: Universal Coverage and Regulated Competitive Markets*. The Commonwealth Fund, New York.

Lijphart A. (1968). *Verzuiling, Pacificatie en Kengtering in de Nederlandse Politiek* ["Pillarization, Pacification and Change in Dutch Politics"]. J. H. de Bussy, Amsterdam.

Maarse H. (2006). "Health Insurance Reform in The Netherlands." Lecture. University of Helsinki, Helsinki.

Maarse H, Okma KGH. (2004). "The Privatisation Paradox in Dutch Health Care." In: Maarse H (ed.), *Privatisation in European Health Care*. Elsevier Gezondheidszorg, Maarssen.

March J, Simon H. (1958). *Organizations*. New York: John Wiley and Sons.

Marmor TR, Okma KGH, Rojas J. (2007). "What It Is, What It Does and What It Might Do: A Review of Michael Moore's *Sicko*." *Am J Bioethics* **7**(10): 49–51.

"Ministerie van Volksgezondheid, Welzijn en Sport" (2008). Accessed 20 October 2008. http://www.minvws.nl

Ministry of Health. (1988). *Verandering Verzekerd* ["Change Assured"]. SDU, The Hague.

Ministry of Health. (1994). *Kostenbeheersing in de Zorgsector* ["Controlling Health Care Expenditures"]. SDU, The Hague.

Ministry of Health. (1996). *Financieel Overzicht Zorg 1997* ["Financial Survey Health Care 1997"]. SDU, The Hague.

Ministry of Health. (2004). *Vraag aan Bod* ["Demand at the Center"]. Ministry of Health, Welfare and Sports, The Hague.

Ministry of Health. (2006). *Rijksbegroting Volksgezondheid, Welzijn en Sport 2007* ["Health Budget 2007"]. Ministry of Health, Welfare and Sports, The Hague.

Ministry of Health. (2007a). "Oplossing Wanbetalersproblementiek (Nominale) Zorgpremie" ["Solution Delinquency Nominal Premiums"]. Letter to Parliament, 12 November. SDU, The Hague.

Ministry of Health. (2007b). "Structurele Aanpak Wanbetalers" ["Structural Solution Delinquents"]. Brief aan TK Over Wanbetalers Zorgverzekering ["Letter to Parliament about Delinquent Payers of Health Insurance"], 23 May. SDU, The Hague.

Naik G. (2007). "Dutch Treatment: In Holland, Some See Model for U.S. Health Care System." *Wall St J*, 6 September.

OECD. (1992). *The Reform of Health Care: A Comparative Analysis of Seven OECD Countries. Health Reform Studies No. 2*. OECD, Paris.

OECD. (1994). *The Reform of Health Care: A Review of Seventeen OECD Countries. Health Reform Studies No. 5*. OECD, Paris.

Okma KGH. (1997a). *Studies in Dutch Health Politics, Policies and Law*. Ph.D. thesis. University of Utrecht, Utrecht.

Okama KGH. (1997b). "Concurrentie, Markten en Marktwerking in de Gesondheidszorg" ["Competition and Markets in Health Care"]. *Themanummer Marktwerking* **20**(2): 164–178.

Okma KGH. (2001). *Health Care, Health Policies and Health Care Reform in The Netherlands*. Ministry of Health, Welfare and Sports, The Hague.

Okma KGH. (2002). "Health Care and the Welfare State: Two Worlds of Welfare Drifting Apart?" In: Berghman J *et al.* (eds.), *Social Security in Transition*. Kluwer Law International, Leiden.

Okma KGH. (2008). "Revenue Changes in Dutch Health Insurance: Individual Mandate or Social Insurance?" The Annual Meeting of the National Academy of Social Insurance. Washington, DC, 31 January–1 February. www.nasi.org

Okma KGH, De Roo AA. (forthcoming). "From Polder Model to Modern Management in Dutch Health Care." In: Marmor TR, Freeman R, KGH Okma (eds.), *Comparative Studies and the Politics of Modern Medical Care*. Yale University Press, New Haven.

Okma KGH, Van der Burg H. (2004). "Das Budgetmodell der Niederländischen Krankenkassen" ["Budgeting Dutch Sickness Funds"]. *Die BBk. Zeitschrift der Betrichlichen Krankenversicherung* **92**(1): 36–39.

Okma KGH, Ooijens M. (2005). "De Patient Centraal: Zijn de Verenigde Staten ons Voorland?" ["Patient-Centered Care: US Health Care as a Model?"]. *Tijdschrift voor de Sociale Sector*, 26–29 June.

Palmer GR, Short SD. (1989). *Health Care and Public Policy — An Australian Analysis*. The Macmillan Company of Australia, Melbourne.

Pickard S, Sheaff R, Dowling B. (2006). "Exit, Voice, Governance and User-Responsiveness: The Case of English Primary Care Trusts." *Soc Sci Med* **63**(1): 373–383.

Regeerakkoord 1994 ["Governing Manifesto 1994"]. (1994). SDU, The Hague.

Regeerakkoord 1998 ["Governing Manifesto 1998"]. (1998). SDU, The Hague.

Regeerakkoord 2007 ["Governing Manifesto 2007"]. (2007). Accessed 29 May 2007. www.regering.nl

Rengers M, Van Uffelen X. (2005). "Het Zorgstelsel is een Sigaar Uit Eigen Doos" ["The Health System as a Dutch Treat"]. *Volksrant*, 22 October.

Rosenberg E. (2006). "Ziekenhuizen Moeten Hard Zijn" ["Hospitals Must Be Hard"]. *NRC Handelsblad,* 18 January.

Rosenberg E. (2007). "Concurrentie in de Zorg Blijft Uit" ["Competition in Health Care Does Not Materialize"]. *NRC Handelsblad*, 15 May.

Scheerder R. (2005). "Kostenbeleid 2005" ["Cost Control Policy in 2005"]. *Zorg & Financiering* **193**(2): 8–28.

Schut FT. (1997). *Competition in Dutch Health Care*. Ph.D. thesis. Erasmus University, Rotterdam.

Schut FT, Van de Ven WPMM. (2005). "Rationing and Competition in the Dutch Health-Care System." *Health Econ* **14**: S59–S74.

Smit M, Mokveld P. (2007). *Verzekerdenmobiliteit en Keuzegedrag* ["Mobility and Choice in Dutch Health Insurance"]. Zeist: Vektis.

Strategisch Akkoord 2002 ["Governing Manifesto 2002"]. (2002). SDU, The Hague.

"Tandarts Terug in Het Basispakket" ["Dental Care Back in Basic Insurance"]. (2007). Accessed 26 May 2007. www.regering.nl

Tuohy CH. (1999). *Accidental Logics: The Dynamics of Change in the Health Care Arena in the United States, Britain, and Canada*. Oxford University Press, New York.

Van de Ven WPMM, Schut FT. (2008). "Universal Mandatory Health Insurance in The Netherlands: A Model for the United States?" *Health Affairs* **27**(3): 771–781.

Van het Loo M, Kahan JP, Okma KGH. (1998). "Recent Developments in Health Care Costs Containment in The Netherlands." In: Mossialos E, Le Grand J (eds.), *Health Care and Cost Containment in the European Union*. Ashgate, Aldershot.

Visser J, Hemerijck A. (1997). *A Dutch Miracle — Job Growth, Welfare Reform and Corporatism in The Netherlands*. Amsterdam University Press, Amsterdam.

Wilensky H. (2002). *Rich Democracies: Political Economy, Public Policy, and Performance*. University of California Press, Berkeley.

"Zorgverzekeraars Nederland" (2008). Accessed 20 October 2008. www.zn.nl

Chapter 3

Reform and Re-reform of the New Zealand System

Toni Ashton[*,†] *and Tim Tenbensel*[†]

Introduction

New Zealand has attracted widespread international attention following a highly ambitious and seemingly radical program of health reform initiated in the 1990s. Less well known, but equally significant, have been the attempts in the 2000s to "re-reform" the health system. Both sets of reforms were driven largely by the ideology of the major political party in government at the time. In spite of these waves of reform, some key aspects of the system have remained remarkably stable and many continuities have endured throughout the reform period (Gauld, 2001; Ashton *et al.*, 2005). The New Zealand experience therefore provides a fascinating case study about the politics of health care, about the resilience of institutions, and about the rhetoric and reality of health sector reform.

The next section provides a brief overview of the structure of the New Zealand health system. This is followed by a description of the waves of reform that have occurred over the past 20 years and the theories and ideas that underpinned them. We then explore some of the drivers (institutions, interests, and values) that have shaped the reforms. Finally,

* Corresponding author.
† School of Population Health, University of Auckland, Private Bag 92D19, Auckland, New Zealand.

we consider the effects that the reforms have had on various dimensions of the system, including funding, governance, patient voice, and choice.

The New Zealand Health System

New Zealand lies at the bottom of the world in the south western Pacific Ocean, approximately 2000 km to the southeast of Australia. Its land area is similar in size to Japan and the United Kingdom, and yet its population is only 4.2 million. About 70% of the population live in the main urban areas, with one third living in the largest city, Auckland. In contrast, around 10% live in remote rural regions. About 67% of the population are of European descent, while 15% identify themselves as Māori (the indigenous people of New Zealand), 9% as Asians, and 7% as Pacific Islanders (Statistics New Zealand, 2008).

The country has a unicameral parliamentary system that historically elected representatives via a first-past-the-post electoral system following the British tradition. A referendum in 1993 led to this system's replacement in 1996 by mixed member proportional representation. Another important feature of New Zealand's constitution is the Treaty of Waitangi, signed between the British Crown and Māori tribes in 1840. This agreement gave Māori the same rights and privileges as British citizens in return for their sovereignty. Although largely ignored until the 1970s, the Treaty of Waitangi now has great influence over both the direction and the process of health policy.

The foundations of New Zealand's public health system were laid through the Social Security Act of 1938, when the government of the day attempted to introduce a universal, fully funded national health system as part of a broader set of welfare reforms. Resistance from medical practitioners who did not wish to become government employees resulted in the emergence of a dual system where hospitals provide services free of charge in state owned hospitals while primary health services fall under private ownership and only receive part of their income from public funds. Although the basket of services covered by public funding expanded significantly in the early years, this basic structure of funding and provision has remained relatively unchanged since its inception.

In 2006, New Zealand spent NZ$15.4 billion (US$10.3 billion), or 9.4% of the GDP, on health care (Ministry of Health, 2008). Seventy-eight percent of this expenditure was from public sources, 17% was out-of-pocket spending, and 5% came from private health insurance. The large majority of public funding comes from general taxation. However, 9% of public funding is accounted for by the Accident Compensation Commission (ACC), a statutory state-owned insurance organization that provides compulsory, comprehensive no-fault insurance cover for accident-related injuries occurring in New Zealand. Funding for the ACC comes from levies paid by employers, employees, the self-employed, and motor vehicle licensing. The ACC also receives some direct funding from the government to cover nonworkers (Ministry or Health, 2007).

All permanent residents in New Zealand are automatically covered by the public health system and receive most services free of charge. This includes inpatient and outpatient health care in state-owned hospitals, maternity services, and many community-based services. Copayments apply for general practice consultations and pharmaceuticals; access to some disability support services (such as home care and long term residential care for older people) is means-tested.

The majority of general practitioners (GPs) in New Zealand work in group practices comprising three or more GPs, one or more practice nurses, and a number of other support staff. Citizens can choose their own provider at the primary care level. However, access to secondary care requires a GP referral, and patients usually have little or no choice of specialist or hospital in the public system. New Zealanders generally perceive waiting lists for nonurgent care to be a problem, although waiting times have reduced significantly in recent years. Long waiting times have, in part, led to the development of a parallel private system in which people can effectively exit the public system and elect to pay for their own care from a private specialist or private hospital of their choice. They pay for that care either from voluntary private health insurance or directly out-of-pocket. About one third of the population hold private health insurance. Private insurance is not subject to any special regulations, and premiums are not tax-deductible.

The system represents a mix of the OECD's "integrated" and "contract" models (OECD, 1992). The Ministry of Health has devolved the vast majority of tax funding to 21 District Health Boards (DHBs) via a weighted population-based funding formula.[1] DHBs are responsible for improving, promoting, and protecting the health and independence of their populations by either providing or purchasing services for the people residing in their geographically defined region (New Zealand Public Health and Disability Act 2000, s22). The DHB "provider arms", as they are called, own the public hospitals and provide hospital services plus some community-based services. DHBs, the ACC, and the Ministry of Health purchase all other services — including most primary health services — from private providers through contracts, or "Service Agreements" (Fig. 1).

Successive Health Reform Waves in New Zealand

Political and Economic Context

The period between 1984 and 1996 witnessed enormous changes in New Zealand's economic policy and public sector management, instigated by both major political parties when in government. Many commentators considered these economic and public sector reforms to be the "purest" translation into practice of neoliberal policy prescriptions and new public management ideas (Boston *et al.*, 1996; Pollitt and Bouckaert, 2000). However, in the period before 1990, the Labour government of the time did not extend such reforms into the arenas of health and social services, perhaps because this would have exposed deep rifts within the party. After this government was swept from office in 1990, the incoming National Party government had fewer qualms about extending the neoliberal reform agenda to the health sector. However, in 1996, its capacity to reform was weakened by the need to coalesce with minor political parties

[1] The Ministry has retained responsibility for public health services, maternity services, and disability support services for people aged under 65 years of age, and purchases this care directly from providers.

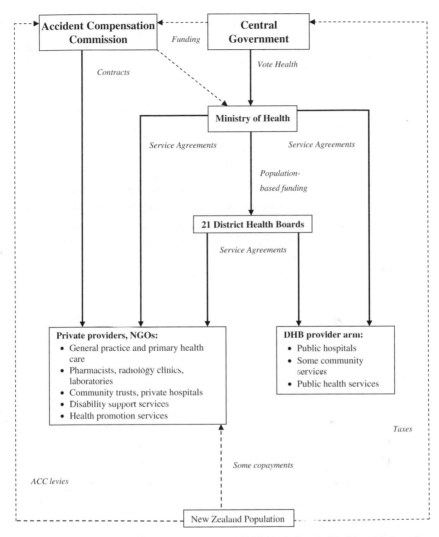

Source: Ministry of Health, 2006, *The Annual Report 2005/06 Including the Health and Independence Report*. Wellington: Ministry of Health.

Fig. 1. Structure of the New Zealand health and disability system.

following the first election under proportional representation. The introduction of proportional representation itself was a consequence of popular discontent with the content, scope, and speed of policy changes that took place under the first-past-the-post electoral system. Consequently,

Table 1. Timeline of Major Reforms

Year(s)	Type of Reform
1938	Social Security Act established legislation for introduction of a universal tax-funded health system
1940s	Introduction of full public funding for hospital and mental health services, and partial funding for a range of primary health services
1983–89	Fourteen Area Health Boards established
1991	Area Health Boards dismissed
1993	Contract model introduced: four Regional Health Authorities established, public hospitals commercialized and renamed Crown Health Enterprises
1997	• Purchasing centralized under Health Funding Authority (HFA) • Crown Health Enterprises restructured and renamed Hospital and Health Services • Free GP consultations and pharmaceuticals for children under six years of age
2000	• Return to a mix of contract and integrated models • HFA abolished • Twenty-one District Health Boards established to purchase and/or provide services for people in their district
2002–07	• Development of 82 Primary Health Organizations • Subsidies for GP consultations and pharmaceuticals increased and made universal

the coalition watered down the reforms and made incremental adjustments during the latter half of the 1990s. Finally, at the turn of the millennium, the incoming center-left government reversed many of the reforms of the 1990s and embarked on its own program of restructuring the health system, with a focus on primary health care.

1980s

As in other high-income countries, the perceived inefficiency of the health system had become a pre-eminent concern in New Zealand by the 1980s. Prior to the 1980s, locally elected hospital boards provided public hospital services and some community-based services while primary health services, disability support services, and public health services received separate funding from central government departments. The highly decentralized system of hospital governance was widely recognized as problematic.

Towards the middle of the 1980s, the government transformed the local hospital boards into 14 Area Health Boards (AHBs) which received global (population-based) budgets. While primary health services (and disability support services) continued to receive separate funding from the central government, the AHBs became responsible for public health services (French *et al.*, 2001). Population-based funding, together with the devolution of funding for public health services, aimed to encourage the AHBs to shift their focus away from the expansion of hospital services towards the development of programs addressing broader public health issues (Gauld, 2001).

The introduction of AHBs was fraught with difficulties, not least because of the problems associated with redressing historical inequities in funding across the regions. The last 4 of the 14 AHBs were finally established in 1989. However, the system was to be short-lived. In 1988, a government-appointed task force drew attention to the problems faced by the public hospitals, particularly the lack of incentives for efficiency and poor accountability mechanisms associated with the integrated model (Gibbs *et al.*, 1988). This report recommended the creation of an organizational split between purchasing and provision. However, the government did not take up the recommendations. At this time, there were considerable tensions within the Labour Party between the neoliberal reformers and the traditional social democrats. Consolidation and amalgamation of hospital boards into AHBs therefore continued as the main direction in health care reform between 1983 and 1990.

Early 1990s: The Big Bang

Just over six months after it was elected to office in late 1990, the incoming National (center-right) government announced plans for a radical restructuring of the public health system (Upton, 1991). These proposals reflected the market-oriented reforms that had been introduced into other sectors of the economy during the 1980s. In July 1991, on the same night that the new government announced the reforms, it summarily dismissed the elected and appointed board members of the AHBs, and replaced them with commissioners whose job it was to oversee the implementation of the proposed new structure. The incoming Health Minister had also made it quite clear to the Ministry of Health officials that their advice on health sector matters was not as highly valued as Treasury advice. Since the 1980s, Treasury advice had been heavily shaped by new institutional economics and a public choice framework for policy, both of which emphasized the perils of "provider capture" and the virtues of market-type mechanisms. Treasury favored a policy prescription of functional separation and single-purpose agencies that their minister or board could steer through clear accountability relationships. These structural design principles also dovetailed nicely with the health-specific structural design favored by Alain Enthoven (Jacobs and Barnett, 2000).

Unlike the move to AHBs, which had taken place over a period of years, the 1993 reforms represent a perfect example of a "big bang" style of reform. The central feature of these reforms was a switch from the integrated AHB model towards a contract model that would separate the roles of purchasing and provision of services. All funding for personal (primary, secondary, and tertiary) health services and disability support services was channeled into a single purse. The Ministry of Health then distributed this money to four newly established Regional Health Authorities, whose role was to purchase services on behalf of the people living in their region. On the provider side, the old public hospitals became for-profit businesses, with the Ministers of Health and Finance as their shareholders. Now renamed Crown Health Enterprises (CHEs), the public hospitals were required to compete with private providers for contracts to supply health services. The CHEs were run as commercial enterprises and many hired chief executives from the private sector to import best business practices. The theory behind this "quasi-market" was that its participants would behave in much the same way as buyers and sellers in a competitive market, with providers responding to the preferences of the

RHAs and the most efficient providers winning the contracts. The original proposal also included the option for patients to take their share of public funding to alternative, nongovernment purchasers once the RHAs were fully established. However, this proposal was never implemented, and so the RHAs did not face the pressures imposed by the potential exit of patients and service users.

Apart from a few relatively minor modifications during the implementation period (Finlayson, 2001), the government implemented the new structure on 1 July 1993, almost two years to the day after it had announced its plans. The expectation of the government was that the new system would:

- Improve access to a health system which is effective, fair, and affordable;
- Encourage efficiency, flexibility, and innovation in health care delivery;
- Reduce waiting times for hospital operations;
- Widen the choice of hospitals and health services for "consumers";
- Enhance the working environment for health professionals;
- Recognize the importance of public health in preventing illness and injury, and in promoting health;
- Increase the sensitivity of the health system to the changing needs of society (Upton, 1991).

By the time of the next general election in 1996, there was little evidence of any major efficiency gains accruing from the new system (Cumming and Salmond, 1998; Ashton, 2002; Easton, 2002). No CHEs had returned any dividends to their two shareholders, and many were in deficit. The agency charged with monitoring the performance of the CHEs concluded that "…the pace of performance seems, if anything, to have declined since the advent of the reforms" (Crown Company Monitoring and Advisory Unit, 1996). This was probably not altogether surprising, given the short time period and the depth and breadth of disruption that the reforms had caused. However, the restructuring had been costly. Moreover, rather than enhancing their working environment, many health professionals felt quite alienated working in a system that encouraged competition between providers (Malcolm *et al.*, 1996). There was also widespread public dissatisfaction with the new system after some services were terminated and after a series of anecdotes wherein patients did not receive adequate care in public hospitals was highly publicized.

Late 1990s: Some Modifications

The 1996 election brought the first coalition government to power, with the National (center-right) party retaining the senior role. The junior partner in the coalition, New Zealand First, was ideologically opposed to a competitive health system. The first health policy statement published by the new government indicated a withdrawal, at least from the rhetoric, of a competitive system. It stated: "The Coalition partners are committed to publicly funded health care that encourages cooperation and collaboration rather than competition between health and disability services.... The new focus [for the CHEs] will be on achieving health outcomes and improving the health status of the populations they serve." (Coalition Government, 1996). And so a new round of restructuring began. While the new government retained the contracting model, it centralized the purchasing responsibilities of the four RHAs under a single national organization, the Health Funding Authority (HFA). The HFA was required to move away from purchasing by competitive tendering and to work more closely with providers in planning service volumes and in establishing benchmark prices. Subsidies for GP consultations and pharmaceuticals were increased for children under six years of age, in order to facilitate free services for young children. On the provider side, CHEs were reconfigured into not-for-profit publicly owned entities called Hospital and Health Services (HHSs). The coalition agreement also limited the extent to which the HFA could purchase services from private hospitals rather than from the HHSs.

2000s: Back to the Future?

At the end of 1999, a new Labour-led coalition government came to power. The Labour Party (the senior coalition partner) was even more opposed to a competitive system than the New Zealand First Party had been in 1996. By this time, the radical neoliberal reformers had broken away from the Labour Party, which had returned to a more traditional social-democratic identity. The Labour Party argued that the previous government had allowed the health system to be "run down, privatized, and corporatized" and that the reforms since 1993 had resulted in "the overwhelming alienation of the public" (New Zealand Labour Party, 1999). It proposed "the restoration of a non-commercial system…" and the "…full involvement of representatives of local communities" in the composition, management, and planning of health services.

Some of this change in direction was linked to a broader program of recasting the public sector reforms of the 1980s and 1990s (Chapman and Duncan, 2007), while other changes reflected a different health policy agenda. The Labour Party had campaigned in 1999 for an end to the mar-ketization and commercialization of health care, and also sought to return to a model of community governance of health, in keeping with the history of New Zealand's hospitals. The incoming government also brought substantive policy objectives such as primary health care reform, improved population health, and reduced health inequalities to the top of the policy agenda.

This led to yet another round of major reform of the health system. The central feature this time around was the establishment of the 21 District Health Boards with locally elected governing bodies. The central purchasing agent (the HFA) was disbanded and its purchasing roles distributed between the DHBs and the Ministry of Health. Although the DHBs share many of the features of the old AHBs, a key point of difference is that the funding envelope of the DHBs includes funding for primary health care and disability support services for those aged 65 years and over. Because private sector organizations provide these services, the DHBs are both providers *and* purchasers of services, and so their roles and responsibilities are much wider than those of the AHBs. While some have argued that a split between purchasing and provision could have worked in concert with greater community input into governance of hospitals (Gauld, 2006), the incoming government opted for community-based governance of both provision *and* purchasing. DHBs were also given greater responsibility for their entire population. This not only required the integration of responsibility for community-based and hospital services within a single organization, but also a strategic planning framework for most publicly funded health services within the district. DHB activities are guided by the New Zealand Health Strategy, which sets out some fundamental principles, goals, and objectives for the sector (King, 2000).

Another important element of this last round of restructuring has been the reform of the primary health care sector. In 2001, the Minister of Health announced the Primary Health Care Strategy, which set out a vision for a primary health system that would focus on the health of populations as well as individuals, was community-oriented, and would encourage a team-based approach to care (King, 2001). The strategy provided substantial financial incentives for the establishment of networks between GPs and other primary health providers in the form of Primary Health Organizations (PHOs). PHOs are nongovernment organizations funded by DHBs on a capitation basis to provide a range of primary health services to their enrolled populations. The health care providers included in PHOs vary, but, in addition to GPs and practice nurses, may include physiotherapists, sexual health clinic workers, dentists, health promotion workers, and other allied health professionals. Although enrolment in PHOs is voluntary, subsidies were increased quite significantly (and hence copayments declined) for patients who joined a PHO. More than 80 PHOs were established within five years, with most GPs and over 95% of the population belonging to a PHO (Ministry of Health, 2007a). The 2006–2010 phase of the Primary Health Care Strategy focuses on reducing inequalities, engaging communities, and improving management of chronic conditions (Ministry of Health, 2007b).

The particular direction and salience of primary health reform is very much a product of the historical development of the primary care sector.

Most importantly, the dual system — in which hospital care was free to users at the point of service, whereas primary care required out-of-pocket payments — produced significant inequities in access to primary care services. It also resulted in high rates of hospitalizations that might have been avoided by better access to ambulatory care. Another driving force of the primary care reforms has been the increased emphasis on improving the health of particular populations.

Summary of the Reform Period

New Zealand stands out as a country that has been ready, willing, and able to make major and frequent changes to the structure and contracting regime of its health system over the past 20 years. Over this period, the prevailing definition of health policy problems has changed substantially, from the need for greater efficiency in the 1980s and 1990s to the need for improvements in population health and reductions in unequal access to health care in the 2000s. As the problem definitions varied, so, too, did the favored policy options of the day, from corporate governance and separation of policy, purchasing, and provision in the 1990s, to devolved democratic governance and a more integrated model (for hospitals) in the 2000s. To use Kingdon's (1984) concepts, the problem, policy, and political streams have not been independent of each other as they are in more complex health systems such as the U.S. Instead, changes in governments result in changes in prevailing problem definitions and policy solutions. Windows of opportunity for change generally open when there is a change of dominant party in government.

In the remainder of this chapter we address two major questions that arise from the New Zealand story. Firstly, what has driven these seemingly dramatic shifts in policy direction over two decades — are such changes attributable to the nature of health policy institutions or has there been fundamental cultural change in New Zealand society? Secondly, to what extent have the results of the reforms lived up to the expectations of those who initiated them?

Drivers of Change

The trajectory of health system reform in New Zealand, as in any national context, is heavily shaped by institutional enablers and constraints, and by underlying cultural values. The factors that matter are New Zealand's particular political system, the entrenched path dependency of tax-based financing, and the dynamics of the state–medical-professional relationship. We argue that, together, these institutional features have been the most influential in shaping the health policy agenda, the speed of change, the accommodation of contending interests, and the character of reform implementation. While cultural values have, on occasions, restricted the introduction and/or implementation of policies, on the whole, major health policy changes appear to have shaped cultural orientations regarding health, rather than vice versa.

Role of the State

The concentrated constitutional power of the New Zealand state, combined with its dominance over health funding and the fact that it is the main provider of hospital services, means that New Zealand governments have more direct levers at their disposal than most other high-income countries. Being predominantly tax-funded, New Zealand's health system is subject to more hands-on control by governments. Constitutional power is highly concentrated (one house of Parliament, unitary system) and this has given the state substantial autonomy. As a result, reforming governments face few formal obstacles and veto points in the pursuit of major policy changes. This single factor explains the comparative ease with which the New Zealand governments of the 1990s and 2000s made significant legislative and structural changes. In contrast to some of the other countries that are featured in this book (such as The Netherlands), where reform has faced numerous constraints, windows of opportunity for major policy reform occur relatively often in New Zealand and tend to stay open for longer than elsewhere.

Such institutional capacity for reform would be the envy of many other high-income countries, yet it clearly has its downside. The concentrated power over policy provides an example of reform "hyperactivity," and carries greater potential for reversal of reforms (Weaver and Rockman, 1993). While some commentators claim that institutional power has been weakened by the move to an electoral system based on proportional representation since 1996, this shift only had a discernible effect on state capacity in the late 1990s. In the 2000s, the main brake on hyperactivity has been a general sense of reform fatigue and a growing realization that structural reform has limited traction.

The high concentration of institutional power also means that novel policy solutions have a much greater chance of adoption due to the absence of veto points. While this facilitates innovation, it can also be problematic — a common feature of all the reforms discussed in this chapter has been a tendency to construct new systems and structures with relatively little consideration of the practicalities of implementation (Gauld, 2008). As such, the waves of reforms have provoked considerable uncertainty and anxiety amongst service providers who were left with the responsibility of translating a broad vision into concrete practice, with very little practical guidance. The 1990s reforms were also noteworthy for the lowered morale of the health providers who experienced the perverse consequences of the competitive model (Malcolm *et al.*, 1996).

It is also important to note that New Zealand governments, whatever their political complexion, have shown no inclination to change from tax-based funding to other forms of financing the health system. The 1991 Taskforce provided the only opportunity in the past two decades to consider moving from a predominantly tax-funded system to an insurance-based system (Upton, 1991). However, there was not sufficient support within the Taskforce, or ultimately within the Cabinet, for such a move (Jacobs and Barnett, 2000). Private insurance as a predominant source of funding never became a serious option, even though it had been strongly advocated in the late 1980s and early 1990s by the Business Roundtable, a group of business leaders who had close links to Treasury and who had been highly influential in other policy areas during the reform period (Goldfinch, 2000).

The Medical Profession

The historical legacy of the dual system of user-pays primary care and publicly funded hospital care has had a profound effect on relations between the state and the medical profession in New Zealand. In effect, it has meant that the policy arenas of primary care and hospitals have been largely separated since the early 1940s. State–doctor relationships in the hospital sector have tended to center on remuneration and the conditions of specialists working as salaried public employees. The existence of a parallel niche private hospital sector, together with an international labor market for their services, allows specialists to exert a high degree of labor market power in their interactions with the state that funds them. As such, the key interest group of medical professionals in the hospital sector, the Association of Salaried Medical Specialists (ASMS), operates essentially as a labor union. Crucially, the specialists used their market power to resist the concerted managerialist push in the 1990s. From the specialists' point of view, however, they are significantly constrained by the level of resources in the public system.

In primary care, the policy territory has been quite different. With the government having lost the battle to prevent GPs from charging copayments in the 1930s, primary care had reverted to a predominantly private industry, with limited state subsidy, between the 1960s and the early 2000s. One major legacy of the 1990s reforms for primary care was the establishment of networks of GPs and other primary health providers. This occurred initially through the formation of Independent Practitioner Associations to offset the power of the RHAs as single purchasers. This organizational development facilitated the establishment of PHOs in the 2000s, which were the mechanism by which the Labour-led coalition government distributed increased public subsidies for primary care. Sensitive to historical concerns of GPs regarding a private business model, fee-for-service payment, and the right to charge copayments, the government opted for a voluntary scheme made sweeter by significant financial incentives. The government also sidelined general practice interest groups from policy formulation in 2000. Nevertheless, the high enrolment in PHOs exceeded the government's most optimistic expectations.

Since the introduction of PHOs in 2002–2006, a dominant concern of GPs has remained the right to set the level of patient fees charged above any government subsidy. While GPs have retained this right, any fees set above a reasonable level are now subject to a review process by DHBs. Thus, this tug of war between the state and the profession now takes place at a local level in negotiations between DHBs and PHOs (and between PHOs and their member doctors). The different policy terrains of primary care and hospitals have meant that interest group activity has tended to be sector-specific, and the New Zealand Medical Association (NZMA) has struggled to find a policy role that is relevant to both general practitioners and hospital specialists.

Cultural Values

Characterizing the cultural values that underlie New Zealand's health system is not a straightforward task. At first glance and in terms of Douglas and Wildavsky's framework (1982), it seems that New Zealand is a classic example of a hierarchical collectivist system. There is solidarity to the extent that there is general support for collective financing. Some commentators have also argued that the system reflects a strong tradition of egalitarianism (Blank and Burau, 2004). In recent years, egalitarian themes have returned to the forefront of health policy through the sustained policy focus on reducing health inequalities. However, this policy emphasis is specific to the Labour-led coalition and is not shared by center-right political parties.

At the same time, there are clear elements of individualism in New Zealand's health system. The perpetuation of a dual system for more than 60 years indicates a tolerance for inequitable access to primary care in tandem with strong support for universal access to hospital care. Similarly, the ability to pay privately for secondary services in order to obtain more timely care or to choose one's specialist and hospital also indicates a tolerance for a degree of inequity in secondary services in return for greater individualism. It is unclear whether or not collectivism has weakened (and individualism has strengthened) over the past 20 years. While ownership of private health insurance has declined over the past decade, this may be more in response to price increases than a reflection of any underlying change in cultural preferences. A fair degree of social responsibility has certainly endured in spite of efforts in the 1990s to encourage greater individual responsibility in more general welfare reform. The unpopularity of the market-based reforms in the 1990s also revealed support for a system of health service delivery based upon collaboration rather than on competition.

More generally, New Zealand's culture has been undergoing some important changes in recent decades. In particular, since the 1970s and 1980s there has been a wider recognition of the need to honor the rights of Māoris under the Treaty of Waitangi. At a practical level, the Māori renaissance of that period paved the way for the spectacular growth of Māori health providers in the 1990s, which was also facilitated by the policy shift towards contracting with nongovernment providers at that time. Migration patterns are changing New Zealand's ethnic mix, in tandem with rapid changes in patterns of social and economic behavior. In time, these cultural shifts may stimulate further changes within the health sector.

Summary

In applying Carolyn Tuohy's (1999) framework of structural and institutional dimensions (discussed in Chapter 1), the New Zealand state has stronger structural power than most other high-income countries. As such, there is a greater degree of hierarchical governance in New Zealand compared to most of the other countries in this collection. Unlike many countries (such as The Netherlands and Israel), in New Zealand organized stakeholders do not generally play a major role in shaping health policy. Nevertheless, the medical profession is far from inconsequential. While it can be, and has been, sidelined from policy formulation, it still manages to exercise considerable influence over implementation of reforms. In the 1990s, resistance to the commercialization of the hospital sector was led by doctors (Easton, 1997), and primary care doctors have also been some-what successful in resisting government attempts to alter the private business foundation of general practice in the 2000s (Gauld, 2008). While cultural values do underpin important changes in the delivery of health services, they do not appear to have been key drivers in the major health reforms of the 1990s and 2000s.

Effects of the Reforms

From an international perspective, the scale and frequency of changes to the New Zealand health system seem to indicate that changes to health reform are easier to engineer than in most countries. But did these health reforms achieve the objectives of the governments that introduced them, and what enduring legacies have they left? Each wave of reform has been accompanied by its own distinctive vocabulary. During the 1990s, the language of markets and competition prevailed (such as purchasers, providers, consumers, and chief executives). In the 2000s, this was replaced with a language more suited to the public sector (hospitals, patients, community representation, and collaboration). However, in spite of the rhetoric that has accompanied the succession of reforms introduced over the past 20 years, many of the key features of the New Zealand health system remain unchanged (Gauld, 2001; Ashton *et al.*, 2005). Thus, the reality of reform has often differed markedly from the rhetoric. As observed in the introduction to this book, it is important to distinguish between formally stated government policy and actually implemented change.

Funding

The argument that many features have remained unchanged in spite of the rhetoric of reform applies most particularly to the method of health care financing: taxation has remained the primary source of funding, the ACC remains in place for the funding of accident-related injuries, people still have the choice to take out private health insurance, public hospital services remain free of charge, and copayments still apply for primary health care for most population groups.[2] What *has* changed, however, is the quantum of money that is now going into health care.

Between 1990 and 2006 (the latest year for which official statistics are available), total expenditure on health care increased from 7% to 9.4% of the GDP. Vote Health funding (the share of tax funds allocated to the Ministry of Health) increased in real terms by 70% between 1996 and 2006 (MoH, 2008). In spite of this, the proportion of public health expenditure has remained fairly stable, at around 77–79% of the total health expenditure (MoH, 2008).

The increase in public funding has, in part, been a deliberate policy by the Labour-led government to expand its investment in the public health system, especially in primary health care. As part of the Primary Health Care Strategy, it gradually increased subsidies for GP consultations and pharmaceuticals between 2001 and 2007. This caused a decline in patient copayments and led to increased utilization rates (Cumming and Gribben, 2007). The government also provided additional funding towards salary increases for health professionals working in public hospitals in an effort to stem the outward migration of trained personnel.

While doctors working in public hospitals continue to receive salaries, most GPs now receive the government subsidy in the form of a capitation payment rather than fees-for-service. In theory, this should encourage greater use of other members of the primary health care team and lead to increased provision of preventive care. However, GPs receive their income from a variety of different sources in addition to the government subsidy. Both the ACC and patients continue to pay a fee for each consultation. There are also special incentive payments for particular services. Any potential impact of capitation on provider behavior is therefore tempered by these other sources of revenue.

---

[2] The National Party government attempted to introduce charges for hospital services in 1992. However, it abolished charges for inpatients just 13 months later, and eliminated the outpatient charges in 1997. In addition, from July 1999, people had the option to choose a private insurance company instead of the ACC for their accident insurance. But this policy was also short-lived: it was abolished after only a few months by the incoming Labour Government in 1999.

Competition and Choice

As far as competition and patient choice are concerned, it is probably fair to say that the 1993 reforms had less impact than the government expected. While providers perceived that there was sometimes strong competition for contracts, most contracts were in fact let to incumbent providers. Most public hospitals continued to enjoy a monopoly in their areas, especially for the provision of acute services. While some private specialists and hospitals did win a few contracts for specified services, private hospitals provided only 1.5% of publicly funded case-mix adjusted discharges in 1999 (MoH, 2000).

The expectation in 1993 was that public hospitals would compete with each other for contracts. However, similar to the experience of other countries that introduced "purchaser–provider splits" (such as the United Kingdom and The Netherlands), the ability to compete was constrained by the need to continue to provide local services to local populations. An analysis of market concentration in New Zealand showed that for a selection of seven common surgical procedures, the degree of market concentration was high both before and after the 1993 reforms (Ashton and Press, 1997). Patient choice of hospitals has therefore remained limited throughout the reform period. In any case, there has been little overt public agitation for increased choice at this level of care.

In sharp contrast to the 1993 reforms, one of the objectives of the 2001 reforms was to *reduce* competition between providers, and "...to avoid routine contestability for hospital services" (New Zealand Labour Party, 1999). Even though competition between providers often seemed more like the wishful thinking of politicians or policy-makers than reality during the 1990s, early analysis for the post-2001 period suggests that collaboration is now increasing both amongst service providers and amongst DHBs as purchasers (Ashton *et al.*, 2008).

As far as primary health care is concerned, there has always been a fairly high degree of competition amongst GPs, and most patients have a choice of provider. The 2001 reforms may have strengthened the power of patient "exit" because PHOs lose the capitation payment when a person decides to switch to another PHO. On the other hand, switching between providers opens up the possibility of risk selection by PHOs and this could dilute the power of exit. As yet, however, not many patients sign up with another PHO, and there is no evidence of systematic selection of low-risk patients by PHOs.

Governance and Voice

A central feature of all four waves of reform has been a shift in the locus of decision-making, with a trend towards increased centralization (from 29 hospital boards to 14 Area Health Boards, to 4 Regional Health Authorities, to 1 Health Funding Authority) during the 1980s and 1990s, followed by a shift back to decentralized decision-making through the 21 District Health Boards in 2001. As the administrative structures changed, so, too, did the methods of governance. In the late 1980s, the long-standing tradition of locally elected boards was maintained for AHBs, although the Minister could supplement the elected board members with up to five appointees to ensure that each board had the required range of skills. Any sense of "voice" at the local level was removed in 1993 when commercial governance arrangements replaced elected boards. Under these arrangements, the expectation was that exit would replace voice as a mechanism for encouraging good provider performance. However, as noted above, in practice, the degree of competition for hospital services was very limited indeed.

In the mid- to late 1990s, the Coalition Government partially withdrew from the fully commercial model and included appointed community representatives on the boards of public hospitals. In 2001, governance arrangements that had prevailed under the AHBs (with boards comprising seven elected members plus up to four more members appointed by the Minister of Health) were reintroduced, so that both voice and decentralized decision-making have now been restored.

Two questions arise from these changing governance arrangements. First, to what extent does devolution of funds actually result in decentralized decision-making? Second, do elected boards result in greater responsiveness to community preferences? In a decentralized system that is funded by central taxes, there will inevitably be tension between the center, which is responsible for raising the money, and the local organizations responsible for spending it. A study of the 2001 reforms in New Zealand during the implementation period found some evidence of such tension: "...a majority of Board members reported that they did not have the level of autonomy necessary to be effective and there were specific reports of 'interference.' In general the role of the centre in policy-making was regarded positively, but there was also a view that local policy decisions were constrained and that central direction extended inappropriately into operational areas" (Barnett and Clayden, 2005).

In attempting to answer the second question, Ashton *et al.* (2005) concluded: "The ability of DHBs to respond to the preferences of their local electorates is likely to be severely curtailed". Reasons for this include the need to comply with national strategies, tight budget constraints, and the difficulties of engaging with local communities in a meaningful way (Tenbensel *et al.*, 2008). Overall, the swings between local and central decision-making that have occurred in New Zealand over the last 20 years, together with the swings between corporate and community governance, are themselves perhaps an indication of the difficulty of striking a balance between being responsive to community preferences and being fiscally accountable.

Conclusion

New Zealand, more than other countries represented in this book, has undergone a series of fairly radical and rapid reforms to its public health system. Perhaps the most obvious explanation for this is the nature of the political institutions. Its unicameral parliament and the absence of federalism mean that governments can bypass opposition from organized stakeholders more easily, and translate policy ideas into actual policy more quickly. Kingdon's (1984) three streams of problems, policies, and politics are therefore not as independent of each other as in more complex institutional systems, and windows of opportunity for reform arise more frequently. However, there was a long period in New Zealand's history (the 1940s to the early 1980s) when governments attempted few major reforms. Why, then, did the period from 1984 to 2002 witness so many changes?

New Zealand, as an English-speaking higher-income country, felt the influence of neoliberal policy prescriptions more strongly and earlier than continental European countries. This influence was accentuated by a sense of economic crisis in the 1980s that prompted political parties to promote more radical policy options. Yet, these neoliberal prescriptions faced more active resistance from professional stakeholders and the public in the health sector than in other policy arenas. In effect, health policy became the key site of an ideological battle between the advocates of market signals and disciplines, and the defenders of a more social-democratic framework in health care.

Accordingly, the two major reforms of the past 20 years were both driven primarily by the political ideology of the government of the day rather than by any careful analysis of policy options. In 1993, the change to a contract model was based upon a belief in the power of markets to achieve efficiency gains. The underlying idea was that "exit" would be the main mechanism driving performance. In contrast, in 2000, the shift back to a more integrated system that featured community governance was based upon the notion that the "voice" of the community would ensure responsiveness to the needs and preferences of the people. In both cases, there was little evidence to support spending large amounts of public money on restructuring the health care system.

Throughout this chapter we have drawn attention to the fact that in New Zealand the reality of the reform has differed from the rhetoric, and that many elements of the system have endured. Although the broad administrative structures changed several times over, the method of financing and many of the underlying organizational arrangements for service delivery remained largely unchanged. This indicates the remarkable resilience of the institutions that drive the health system, even in the face of concerted attempts by governments to transform the delivery of services and entitlements (Pierson, 1994).

In spite of some fundamental differences in political ideology, the two major political parties agree on the need for stability in the overall organizational arrangements of the health system. There will, however, inevitably be incremental adjustments to the current structure as well as ongoing local innovations to service delivery. While reform efforts in New Zealand have concentrated primarily on the whole-system structural changes, it may be that local innovations have a greater impact on system performance and patient outcomes than top-down structural change.

Thus, New Zealand's contribution to the comparative study of health policy is its demonstration of some important limits of health policy reform. It shows what can happen when the "irresistible force" of political institutions that facilitate major policy change meets the "immovable object" of a highly path-dependent health sector. The end result is that major changes occur frequently, but the effects of these changes tend to be far less than hoped for by the governments that initiate them.

References

Ashton T. (2002). "Running on the Spot: Lessons from a Decade of Health Reform in New Zealand." *Appl Health Econ Health Policy* **1**(2): 97–106.

Ashton T, Press D. (1997). "Market Concentration in Secondary Health Services Under a Purchaser–Provider Split: The New Zealand Experience." *Health Econ* **6**: 13.

Ashton T, Mays N, Devlin N. (2005). "Continuity Through Change: the Rhetoric and Reality of Health Reform in New Zealand." *Soc Sci Med* **61**(2): 253–262.

Barnett P, Clayden C. (2005). *Governance in District Health Boards 2002–2005: Report for the 2001 District Health Boards Evaluation Project.* Health Services Research Centre, Victoria University, Wellington. Accessed 28 November 2008. http://www.victoria.ac.nz/hsrc/reports/downloads/Report%20No.%202 %20Governance.pdf.

Blank R, Burau V. (2004). *Comparative Health Policy.* Palgrave MacMillan, New York.

Chapman J, Duncan G. (2007). "Is There Now a New 'New Zealand Model'?" *Pub Management Rev* **9**(1): 1–25.

Coalition Government. (1996). *Policy Area: Health.* Coalition Government, Wellington.

Coney S. (1996). "Political Prognosis." *Sunday Star-Times*, 15 September.

Crown Company Monitoring and Advisory Unit. (1996). *Crown Health Enterprises: Briefing to the Incoming Minister.* Crown Company Monitoring and Advisory Unit, Wellington.

Cumming J, Gribben B. (2007). *Evaluation of the Primary Health Care Strategy: Practice Data Analysis 2001–2005.* Health Services Research Centre, Wellington.

Cumming J, Salmond G. (1998). "Reforming New Zealand Health Care." In: Ranade W (ed.), *Markets and Health Care: A Comparative Analysis.* Addison-Wesley Longman, New York.

Douglas M, Wildavsky A. (1982). *Risk and Culture.* University of California Press, Berkeley.

Easton B. (1997). *The Commercialisation of New Zealand.* Auckland University Press, Auckland.

Easton B. (2002). "The New Zealand Health Reforms of the 1990s in Context." *Appl Health Econ Health Policy* **1**(2): 107–112.

Finlayson M. (2001). "Policy Implementation and Development." In: Davis P, Ashton T (eds.), *Health and Public Policy in New Zealand.* Oxford University Press, Auckland.

French S, Old A, *et al.* (2001). *Health Care Systems in Transition: New Zealand.* European Observatory on Health Care Systems, Paris.

Gauld R. (2001). *Revolving Doors: New Zealand's Health Reforms.* Institute of Policy Studies, Wellington.

Gauld R. (2006). "Health Policy and the Health System." In: Miller R (ed.), *New Zealand Government and Politics*, 4th ed. Oxford University Press, Auckland.

Gauld R. (2008). "The Unintended Consequences of New Zealand's Primary Health Care Reforms." *J Health Polit Policy Law* **33**(1): 93–115.

Gibbs A, Fraser D, Scott J. (1988). *Unshackling the Hospitals: Report of the Hospital and Health Related Services Taskforce.* Hospital and Health Related Services Taskforce, Wellington.

Goldfinch S. (2000). *Remaking Economic Policy*. Victoria University Press, Wellington.

Jacobs K, Barnett P. (2000). "Policy Transfer and Policy Learning: A Study of the 1991 New Zealand Health Services Taskforce." *Governance* **13**(2): 185–213.

King A. (2000). *The New Zealand Health Strategy*. Ministry of Health, Wellington.

King A. (2001). *The Primary Health Care Strategy*. Ministry of Health, Wellington.

Kingdon J. (1995). *Agendas, Alternatives, and Public Policies*. 2nd ed. Harper Collins College Publishers, New York.

Malcolm L, Barnett P, *et al.* (1996). "Lost in the Market? A Survey of Senior Public Health Service Managers in New Zealand's Reforming Health System." *Austr NZ J Pub Health* **20**(6): 567–573.

Ministry of Health. (2000). *Hospital Throughput Statistics 1998/99*. Ministry of Health, Wellington.

Ministry of Health. (2006). *The Annual Report 2005/06 Including the Health and Independence Report*. Ministry of Health, Wellington.

Ministry of Health. (2007a). "Primary Health Care." Accessed 27 November 2008. http://www.moh.govt.nz/moh.nsf/indexmh/phcs-pho

Ministry of Health. (2007b). "Primary Health Care: Implementation Programme 2006–2010: Primary Workings — Issue 3, June 2007." Accessed 27 November 2008. http://www.moh.govt.nz/moh.nsf/ indexmh/phcs-iwp-newsletter-jun07#phofunding.

Ministry of Health. (2008). *Health Expenditure Trends in New Zealand 1996–2006*. Ministry of Health, Wellington.

New Zealand Labour Party. (1999). *Focus on Patients: Labour on Health*. New Zealand Labour Party, Wellington.

OECD. (1992). *The Reform of Health Care: A Comparative Analysis of Seven OECD Countries*. OECD, Paris.

Pierson P. (1994). *Dismantling the Welfare State: Reagan, Thatcher and the Politics of Retrenchment*. Cambridge University Press, Cambridge.

Pollitt C, Bouckaert G. (2000). *Public Management Reform: A Comparative Analysis*. Oxford University Press, London.

Select Committee Report. (2007). "2007/08 Estimates for Vote Health." Accessed 27 November 2008. http://www.parliament.nz/en-NZ/SC/Reports/b/3/5/48DBSCH_SCR3837_1-2007-08-Estimates-for-Vote-Health.htm.

Statistics New Zealand. (2008). "QuickStats about Culture and Identity." Accessed 27 November 2008. http://www.stats.govt.nz/census/ 2006-census-data/quickstats-about-culture-identity/quickstats-about-culture-and-identity.htm?page=para002Master

Tenbensel T, Cumming J, *et al.* (2008). "Where There's a Will, Is There a Way?: Is New Zealand's Publicly Funded Health Sector Able to Steer Towards Population Health?" *Soc Sci Med* **67**(7): 1143–1152.

Tuohy CH. (1999). *Accidental Logics: The Dynamics of Change in the Health Care Arena in the United States, Britain and Canada.* Oxford University Press, New York.

Upton S. (1991). *Your Health and the Public Health.* Ministry of Health, Wellington.

Weaver RK, Rockman B (eds.) (1993). *Do Institutions Matter? Government Capabilities in the United States and Abroad.* Brookings Institute, Washington.

Chapter 4

Health Care Reforms in Singapore

*Meng-Kin Lim**

Introduction

The Republic of Singapore is a tiny island-state of 700 sq km and 4.5 million people, one of the most densely populated countries in the world. Founded in 1819 as a British colonial outpost, it gained self-rule from Britain in 1959 and independence from Malaysia in 1965. It is a parliamentary democracy. The ruling People's Action Party (PAP) has been in power since 1959, and thus has had the rare advantage of being able to pursue its reform agenda without much opposition or undue interruption. Furthermore, economic growth over the past three decades has averaged 8% annually, which makes for a favorable starting point for implementing health care reforms.

Singapore inherited from the British a largely tax-based public health care system, but the standards were basic and rudimentary. To fulfill an election pledge to "bring health care closer to the people," the government decentralized primary care in 1960. Primary care shifted from one main overcrowded General Hospital, which was registering 2400 outpatient visits daily, to 26 satellite outpatient clinics and 46 maternal and child health clinics scattered throughout the island — a task that took four years to accomplish. But apart from this, little else changed. As the Health Minister candidly explained in 1967, "health would rank, at most, fifth in order of priority for funds — after national security, job creation, housing,

* Department of Epidemiology & Public Health, Yong Loo Lin School of Medicine, National University of Singapore.

and education, in that order" (Yong, 1967). And so health care reform languished on the back burner for the next 20 years.

It was not until the mid-1980s, when Singapore had emerged as one of Asia's economic miracles, and when housing, education, job security, and other basic needs had been met in good measure, that the health care system underwent a major overhaul. The principal driver for health care reform was the rising aspirations of the people accompanying their newly found affluence. But for a government that was elected in 1959 on a democratic socialism platform, a very unorthodox theme was chosen as the centerpiece of its reform plan: the 1983 National Health Plan emphasized "individual responsibility" and "co-payment," even as it outlined an ambitious 20-year plan to modernize health care facilities and raise medical standards. The same no-nonsense, "no free lunch" approach, which had underpinned Singapore's almost single-minded pursuit of economic growth, would be applied to health care. The government felt that welfarism was not a viable option, as it bred dependency on the state. It thus adopted a policy of co-payment to encourage the population to assume personal responsibility for their own welfare. In practice, this approach meant the use of pricing to curb demand while simultaneously softening the consequences to protect lower income groups.

Singapore has indeed achieved a great deal in a short period. Its health indicators now compare favorably with the best in the world. Patients have complete free choice of providers. Private providers, some listed on the Stock Exchange, account for 20% of inpatient beds and 80% of outpatient visits. The government publishes comparative lists of procedure prices at different hospitals and selected quality indicators to empower consumers. Market competition is encouraged, health tourism is actively promoted and Singapore is well on its way to attaining medical hub status in Asia.

Health Care Financing

Health care financing is premised on the principle of cost-sharing. The key reforms were Medisave (1984), MediShield (1990), and Medifund (1993). Medisave is an individual medical savings account designed in such a way as to encourage consumer prudence while fostering family solidarity. Medisave is supplemented by Medishield, an in-case-of-catastrophe health insurance scheme that protects households from large and unexpected financial losses. Medifund is a state funded safety net, which takes care of the poor and needy.

Medisave

Medisave was introduced as an extension of the Central Provident Fund (CPF), a save-as-you-earn pension savings scheme started by the British colonial government in 1955 and left intact following Singapore's independence because of its consistency with the government's development strategy, which emphasized high levels of savings and investment. In the years since, CPF has evolved into a comprehensive social security savings scheme that not only caters to members' retirement needs, but also allows for pre-retirement withdrawals to purchase homes and buy home mortgage insurance. Members can even use Medisave to invest in "blue chip" stocks and pay for their children's college expenses. But the core features of the scheme have not changed since its inception: it is compulsory for all employees or self-employed persons who are Singapore citizens or permanent residents, tax-exempt, and interest-yielding. The government guarantees a minimum risk-free interest of 2.5%. In 2008, the actual interest earnings were 4%.

Every CPF member has three accounts: an Ordinary Account for buying a home or paying for CPF approved insurance, investments, and education; a Special Account for old age, contingency purposes, and investment in retirement-related financial products (e.g. life annuity); and a Medisave Account for hospitalization expenses (including convalescent hospitals and hospice care), certain expensive outpatient treatments (like day-surgery, radiotherapy, chemotherapy, renal dialysis, and *in vitro* fertilization), and approved medical insurance.

CPF is not unique to Singapore. It was implemented elsewhere in Britain's colonies, including British Malaya and Africa, to ensure that the social security needs of the aging populations would not drain British public funds. It is Medisave, the world's first medical savings account, that is unique to Singapore. It represents 6–8% of an individual's wages (depending on age) sequestered in the individual's CPF account and earmarked for the medical benefits of the contributor. There is a small element of risk pooling among family members, as Medisave can be used to pay for the hospitalization and other approved medical bills of one's spouse, children, parents or grandparents. Any unspent balance is passed on to the account holder's beneficiaries upon his or her death (Lim, 2004a). In 2008, the combined Medisave accounts of all Singaporeans amounted to SG$42.4 billion (or US$30.0 billion; 1 Singapore dollar equaled 0.7 US dollars in 2008) — a not insignificant sum considering that in 2005, national health care expenditure amounted to SG$7.4 billion, or 3.7% of gross domestic product (GDP). Of this, government expended only about SG$1.8 billion, or 0.9% of GDP.

Medishield

Medishield is a voluntary, low cost, individual medical insurance scheme designed to help Singaporeans pay for large hospitalization bills in case of unforeseen catastrophe, such as serious illnesses or prolonged hospitalization (see Table 1). Medishield is not compulsory, and operates on an opt-out basis. Medisave funds can be used to pay for the premiums (which range from SG$30 per year for those aged 30 and below to SG$705 for the maximum coverage age of 85, or about US$21 to US$498) of the state-operated Medishield scheme (see Table 2). Singapore classifies public hospital wards based on comfort level (from single bed rooms to open dormitories with eight or more beds); Medishield claims are pegged at the subsidized B2 and C class rates. Singaporeans who prefer greater benefits or wish to enjoy higher classes of wards are free to opt for a variety of enhanced "Shield" plans offered by private insurers. The government requires these "Shield" plans to incorporate the basic MediShield plan as a minimum. There are currently 25 such "integrated" Shield Plans offered by five private insurers, catering to the varied health insurance needs of Singaporeans. Some private Shield Plans no longer place limits on the amount that can be claimed each day for hospital stays and procedures, while others offer riders that pay for the deductible portions of the bill.

Table 1. Medishield Benefits

Benefits	Claim Limits (in SGD)
Inpatient/Day surgery	
Daily ward & treatment charges[a]	$250 per day
Daily ward & treatment charges in intensive care unit (ICU)[a]	$500 per day
Surgical operations[b]	
Table 1	$150
Table 2	$300
Table 3	$600
Table 4	$720
Table 5	$840
Table 6	$960
Table 7	$1100
Implants/approved medical consumables[c]	$2500 per treatment
Radiosurgery treatment[d]	$4800 per procedure
Outpatient treatments[e]	
Stereotactic radiotherapy treatment for cancer	$1000 per treatment
Radiotherapy for cancer:	
— External or superficial	$80 per treatment day
— Brachytherapy with or without external	$160 per treatment day
Chemotherapy for cancer/certain benign neoplasms	$150 per 7-day treatment cycle
	$700 per 21- or 28-day treatment cycle
Renal dialysis	$1000 per month
Erythropoietin drug for chronic renal failure	$200 per month
Immunosuppressant drugs for organ transplant	$200 per month
Maximum claim limits	
Per policy year	$50,000
Lifetime	$200,000
Last entry age	Below 75 when cover commences
Maximum coverage age	85 (age next birthday)

[a] Including meal charges, prescriptions, professional charges, investigations, and other miscellaneous charges. (1 SGD = 0.7 USD)

[b] Surgical operations are classified according to their level of complexity, which increases from Table 1 to Table 7.

[c] Approved medical consumables are:

— intravascular electrodes used for electrophysiological procedures

— percutaneous transluminal coronary angioplasty (PTCA) balloons

— intra-aortic balloons (or balloon catheters).

[d] Radiosurgery includes Novalis radiosurgery and Gamma Knife treatment.

[e] Deductibles are not applicable for Outpatient Treatment.

Table 2.   Annual Medishield Premium Table

Age Next Birthday	Yearly Premium
30 and under	$30
31–40	$40
41–50	$80
51–60	$160
61–65	$225
66–70	$265
71–73	$335
74–75	$375
# 76–78	$420
# 79–80	$510
# 81–83	$600
# 84–85	$705

Hence, a carefully chosen plan could reimburse as much as the entire hospital bill.

Medishield currently covers, on average, 80% of the larger hospital bills for subsidized (B2 or C class) patients. The scheme is periodically reviewed so as to ensure higher payouts to keep up with medical inflation. The number of MediShield policyholders covered in 2006 was 2.75 million (or 78% of Singapore citizens and permanent residents). In 2008, the total MediShield coverage was 3.1 million (or 84%) of the population, with 1.3 million subscribers for the Basic MediShield Plan and 1.8 million for the various enhanced Integrated Shield Plans.

Medifund

The third "M" — Medifund — is the state-funded safety net that takes care of those without the means to pay, including people not covered by Medisave or Medishield, or those who have exhausted their quota in these schemes. Medifund was set up as a large government-sponsored endowment fund. Its interest income is distributed to the public hospitals and voluntary welfare organizations to cover costs of patients genuinely unable to pay their hospital bills. Ability or inability to pay is established through means testing and approval authority is decentralized to various hospitals' Medifund commit-tees. In 2008, the fund stood at SG$1.7 billion (or US$1.2 billion) and the disbursement amounted to SG$74 million (or US$52.4 million).

Mixed, Multi-Layered Funding System

Medisave, Medishield, and Medifund, however, together constitute only a minor component of a mixed and multi-layered health care financing system. Medisave currently accounts for a mere 8% of national health care expendi-ture, while Medishield and Medifund combined account for not more than 2%. The remainder of the health expenditure pie comprises employer bene-fits (35%), government subsidies (25%), out-of-pocket payment (25%), and private insurance (5%). While the thrust of the government's health care financing philosophy is "shared responsibility," at no stage of the health care reform process did the government abrogate its responsibility for the poor and needy because at all times the original taxed-based public safety net held firm. In fact, underpinning Singapore's health care financing reform is a 1993 pledge by the government that "no Singaporean will ever be denied needed health care because of lack of funds" (Lim, 1998). The net result of

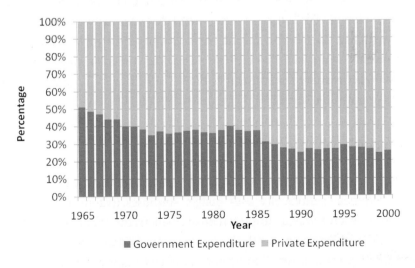

Fig. 1. Government versus private share of total health care expenditure.

Singapore's health care financing reform was a gradual shift of the financial burden from the government to the private sector (Fig. 1), done at a pace and in a manner that the people could bear.

Eldercare Fund and Eldershield

The percentage of the population aged 65 and above is presently 8%, but is projected to reach 25% in 2030. In direct response to concerns about the rapidly aging population, the government has set up a state-funded "Eldercare Fund" in 2000 to provide subsidies to voluntary welfare organizations that offer care to the elderly. This fund is targeted to reach SG$2.5 billion (US$1.8 billion) by 2010. Eldercare was followed in 2002 by the introduction of Eldershield, an affordable insurance scheme for severe disability that provides insurance coverage to those who require long-term care, with premiums payable from Medisave accounts. Eldershield initially provided lifetime coverage for SG$300 (US$212) per month up to a maximum of 60 months (calculated to sufficiently cover a substantial portion of patients' out-of-pocket share of subsidized nursing home care or home care at 2002 prices), it has since been enhanced to meet the varied needs of Singaporeans. It now pays up to SG$400 (US$283) per month, up to a maximum of seventy-two months. The Eldershield Reform of 2007 has allowed Singaporeans who want and are able to afford better coverage to opt for Eldershield Supplements, while the basic Eldershield package remains affordable. More than 4000 people have benefited from Eldershield since its inception in 2002. There are now more than 850,000 Eldershield policy holders.

Affirmative Action

Affirmative action is built into the various schemes as they evolve. Notably, the government periodically uses budget surpluses to top up the various schemes in such a way as to preferentially benefit the less well off and the elderly. For example, in 2001 the government paid two years' worth of MediShield premiums for all Singaporeans aged 61 and above, while setting aside a total of SG$19 million (US$13.4 million) to help the elderly pay for their ElderShield premiums. By 2004, SG$2.75 billion (US$1.9 billion) had gone into the Medisave Top-Up Scheme for the elderly and the Medishield Top Up Scheme for the elderly. In 2008, in order to help older Singaporeans pay for their increased MediShield premiums, the government topped up the Medisave accounts of all those aged 51 and above by up to SG$450 (US$318) per person — this one-time exercise cost the government SG$220 million (US$155 million). The government also topped up the ElderCare Fund by SG$400 million (US$283) in 2008, bringing its size to SG$1.5 billion (US$1.1 billion). It also topped up Medifund by SG$200 million (US$141 million), bringing the fund size to SG$1.7 billion (US$1.2 million).

Targeting of Subsidies

Singapore's graded public hospital ward system is stratified according to level of comfort and amenities; options range from single bed rooms to open dormitories with eight or more beds. Patients in Class A beds pay full costs, while those in Class C enjoy an 80% subsidy. Though patients pay more for higher levels of comfort and improved amenities, there is no difference in the standard of clinical care. The disparities are the result of individual choice. Thus, better distributional outcomes are achieved by treating the majority, who can afford to pay, as co-paying partners and targeting special provisions at the minority who cannot afford to pay. Moreover, the more costly "leveling down" option of ensuring universal access regardless of ability to pay (in which the undeserving rich enjoy the same handouts as the poor) is avoided. The Health Ministry estimates that more than 96% of B and almost 98% of C patients should be able to pay for their bills in full from their Medisave account.

Means Testing to Better Target Subsidies

The Health Ministry has been monitoring hospitalization trends over the years. It recently expressed concern that many who can afford better classes of wards have been choosing to be admitted to the heavily subsidized C and B2 class wards, sometimes crowding out lower income patients. The Health Ministry thus proposed implementing means tesing to determine patients' eligibilty for the heavily subsidized wards. The major obstacle to means testing was the practicality of implementation: What parameters to use? Will the income cut-off points be acceptable to the public? Will implementation be onerous for some? After several years of public dialogue and internal deliberation, the Health Ministry finally announced in 2008 that it would be ready to implement means testing to determine eligibility and the amount of subsidy commencing January 2009.

The cut-off salary for enjoying the full subsidy at public hospitals has been fixed at an income of SG$3200 (US$2265) a month. Using SG $3200 (US$2265) a month as a base, the Health Ministry has produced a detailed sliding scale of declining subsidies according to individual income. In other words, the higher up the salary scale, the smaller the subsidy entitlement (see Table 3). The graduated subsidies are between 50–65% for Class B2 and between 65–80% for Class C. Those earning SG $5201 (US$3681) or more will continue to enjoy a subsidy of 65% in a C class ward and 50% in a B2 class ward. The subsidies for permanent residents who are non-citizens will be 10 percentage points lower than that for citizens. Those with no income, like housewives, retirees, and children, and those living in government-subsidized Housing Board apartments or properties with annual values of SG$11,000 (US$7785) or less, will continue to receive the full subsidy of 80% in C class wards and 65% in B2 class wards. The government estimates that 80% of Singaporeans will hardly be affected by this change. It has promised that the additional revenue derived from the reduced subsidy for the higher income group will go towards subsidizing the lower income group. Patients who cannot afford the current B2 or C subsidy will receive additional financial assistance through Medifund. Persons aggrieved by means testing will have their cases re-assessed on a case-by-case basis. To ensure non-contentious and fuss-free implementation, the government has pledged to be flexible at the margins and "err on the side of generosity."

Health Care Provision

Health care provision comprises seven public hospitals and six specialty centers, which together account for 80% of inpatient beds, with 16 private

Table 3. Means Testing Income Bands and Subsidy Levels

Average Monthly Income of Patient	Class C Subsidy (Citizens) (%)	Class B2 Subsidy (Citizens) (%)	Class C Subsidy (Permanent Residents) (%)	Class B2 Subsidy (Permanent Residents) (%)
$3200 and below	80	65	70	55
$3201–$3350	79	64	69	54
$3351–$3500	78	63	68	53
$3501–$3650	77	62	67	52
$3651–$3800	76	61	66	51
$3801–$3950	75	60	65	50
$3951–$4100	74	59	64	49
$4101–$4250	73	58	63	48
$4251–$4400	72	57	62	47
$4401–$4550	71	56	61	46
$4551–$4700	70	55	60	45
$4701–$4850	69	54	59	44
$4851–$5000	68	53	58	43
$5001–$5100	67	52	57	42
$5101–$5200	66	51	56	41
$5201 and above	65	50	55	40

hospitals accounting for the remaining 20%. Primary health care is easily accessible through an extensive and convenient network of private general practitioners (80%) and public outpatient polyclinics (20%). In addition, an estimated 12% of daily outpatient visits are to Traditional Chinese Medicine (TCM) practitioners in the private sector.

Primary Care

Patients have complete freedom of choice of providers and most go to their own neighborhood family physician — a reflection of the affordability of primary care and a preference for more personalized care. This trend had become evident by the 1980s. By that time, the government had consolidated all its outpatient clinics and maternal and child health clinics (which had become run-down) into 16 ultra-modern polyclinics catering to all age groups. These one-stop centers provide immunization, health promotion activities, health screening, well-women programs, family planning services, nutritional services, psychiatric counseling, dental care, pharmaceuticals, X-ray and laboratory services, and even home-nursing and rehabilitative services for non-ambulatory patients. Charges remain very affordable: SG$8 (US$6) for adults, and SG$4 (US$3) for the elderly (aged 65 and above) and children (under 18 years of age). In comparison, the average consultation fee charged by a private general practitioner is SG$19 (US$13).

Traditional Medicine

Singapore's population is culturally diverse: 77% Chinese, 17% Malay, 8% Indian, and 1% other minority groups. Most originated from China, India, and the Malay Archipelago, and each subpopulation brought its own brand of traditional medicine. Although these medical practices have become "alternatives" to conventional Western medicine, they have over time retained their popularity. Traditional Chinese Medicine (TCM) is the most widely used form of complementary or alternative medicine (88%), followed by Traditional Malay (Jamu) Medicine (8%), and Traditional Indian (Ayuverdic) Medicine (3%). The Ministry of Health estimates that 12% of daily outpatient visits are with TCM practitioners. This fact, coupled with concern for patient safety, motivated the government to enact a system of registration and licensing for TCM practitioners. TCM practitioners are now regulated by a self-regulating body, which is in turn regulated by the Chinese Propriety Medicines Listing Unit in the Ministry of Health.

Secondary and Tertiary Care

Singaporeans are served by a total of 29 well-equipped hospitals and national specialty centers, with 11,545 beds (or 2.6 beds per 1000 Singaporeans). Seven public hospitals and six national specialty centers account for 80% of the beds. The remaining 16 hospitals are privately owned, varying in size from 20 to 505 beds. Competition for patients, who are completely free to choose their health care provider, is keen.

Competition for top talent specialists is even keener. The loss of top specialists to the booming private sector was in fact one of the factors that led to the granting of hospital autonomy in 1985. Freed from civil service constraints, these public sector hospitals could compete with, and set the benchmark for, the private sector. Today, no one bats an eyelid if a top heart surgeon in the public hospitals earns more than US$1 million a year.

This is a far cry from the situation in 1960, when less than 50 doctors in the whole country possessed higher specialist qualifications, and almost all were in public service. To develop the base for tertiary care, beginning from the mid-1970s, the government sent the crème-de-la-crème in the public sector to the best medical centers in the world for training. By the mid-1980s, clusters of private medical specialist clinics were mingling side by side with gleaming shopping malls on Singapore's fashionable Orchard Road, anchored by two private hospitals with tertiary capabilities. Many specialists left the public sector for the lucrative private sector as soon as they made a name for themselves and had served out their government "bonds."

Commercialization of Health Care

Commercialization of medicine is actively encouraged. The major private hospital chains are listed on the stock exchange and are fast expanding into the region, tapping into the booming multi-billion dollar Asian health care markets, estimated to be worth SG$7 billion (US$5.0 billion) in 2010. Foreign patient figures doubled from 200,000 in 2002 to 400,000 in 2005. Four out of five were treated at private clinics and hospitals. Growth in the number of foreign patients has been averaging 20% in the last few years, thanks to stepped-up efforts by Singapore Medicine, a government-industry partnership established in 2003 to turn Singapore into a leading medical hub. Various government agencies work in concert, each playing a distinct role in Singapore Medicine. For example, the Economic Development Board attracts healthcare and biomedical investments, and co-funds developments in high-tech healthcare capabilities. International Enterprise Singapore (known formerly as the Singapore Trade Development Board) supports regionalization of the local healthcare players; the Singapore Tourism Board looks after international marketing and promotes people-oriented services, in collaboration with the Ministry of Health. In August 2006, McKinsey & Company was hired to draw up strategies to help Singapore Medicine attain its goals. The city-state's vibrant biosciences research and development environment also enhances its reputation as a center of medical excellence. Mandatory hospital quality committees and voluntary Joint Commission International (JCI) accreditation ensure that clinical quality and patient safety conform to international standards. In fact, one-third of Asia's JCI accredited health care facilities are to be found in Singapore (Newsweek, 2007).

Domestically, the government has signaled it would like to see the private share of hospital beds in Singapore increase to 30%; it has offered a slew of incentives, including the sale of land sites adjacent to existing public sector hospitals. The government had previously resisted the idea of allowing private hospitals within the campuses of the public hospitals on the ground that Singaporeans might find the overt promotion of private medicine distasteful. But times have changed, and it appears that the government now considers Singaporeans ready. In fact, it rationalizes that such a move will not only attract foreign patients, but benefit Singaporeans as well, since doctors will be able to gain experience treating less common diseases because they are not limited to just local patients.

Hospital Restructuring

The most significant failed health care reform in Singapore's recent history was the attempted privatization of public health care institutions in 1985. The backdrop to this was the economic recession of the mid-1980s, when the government sought to transfer the engine of economic growth from the public to the private sector. A 1986 Report of the Economic Committee had mentioned health care as a prime candidate for deregulation and privatization. An explicitly stated goal was to attract and retain top medical talent in the public sector; once freed of civil service constraints, hospitals could hire and fire at will, and could pay handsome salaries if they wished to. The government considered various models to reduce or eliminate the Ministry of Health's (MoH) control and grant hospitals autonomy. These ranged from a statutory board that would manage public hospitals to wholesale privatization. At first, the government chose the latter. Widespread public unhappiness over the planned privatization, however, led to months of intense debate in public forums, the media, and Parliament. In a rare instance of retreat in the face of negative public opinion, the government modified its original privatization plan, which had entailed wholesale large-scale privatization of hospitals and specialist medical centers. It opted instead for "restructuring," or in World Bank parlance, "corporatization" (Phua, 1991; Preker and Harding, 2003) to achieve the same ends of improving efficiency while reducing state-funded health spending. Each hospital would become an independent entity within the meaning of Singapore's Companies Act and, although remaining 100% government-owned, would be autonomous in fiduciary and operational matters.

The hospital restructuring process took more than 20 years to roll out. The government created a monolithic government company, the Health Corporation of Singapore (HCS) Private Limited in 1987 to own and manage all corporatized hospitals and specialty centers. The independent hospitals, although "private" in name and each governed by its own board of directors, were actually "public" since they were 100% owned by the HCS, which in turn was 100% owned by the government. By 2000, every public hospital and specialist medical center had been restructured, even the largest center — a 2700-bed mental health hospital. As market mechanisms and structures replaced old bureaucratic ones, efficiency and service levels indeed improved. The reforms resulted in raised standards of care and levels of service that were a far cry from the overcrowded wards and unresponsive outpatient clinics of yesteryear. Today, the average waiting time for elective surgery is a mere two weeks while overall patient satisfaction is 80% (Lim, 2004b).

Once restructured, the hospitals were free to set their own directions and to compete with each other. Doctors saw sharp pay rises. But as each hospital focused on its own survival and bottom line, competition became counter-productive. Dysfunctional business tactics were employed, like poaching staff from other hospitals by offering higher salaries. Non-cooperation between institutions resulted in missed opportunities for exploiting economies of scale, such as central drug purchasing and development of a common IT platform for electronic medical records. Each hospital's CEO vied to increase its market share through high-tech acquisitions and other means, confident that the HCS or the MoH would eventually bail them out if they ran deficits. Hospital expenditures rose sharply as a result, contributing to health care cost inflation. There was also concern with over-servicing of patients and inappropriate care, as the new financial incentives designed to retain top specialists in the public sector rewarded doctors according to the volume of procedures performed.

Clustering

The government intervened in 2000. Believing that competition would work better with a smaller number of competitors, it arbitrarily regrouped the restructured institutions into two competing clusters: the National Healthcare Group and the Singapore Health Services. These quasi-independent clusters would still report to the Health Ministry since the Ministry appointed their boards. Simultaneously, the two clusters took control over all the government polyclinics for primary care. Thus in one fell swoop, government achieved horizontal and vertical integration of all public sector health care providers at the primary, secondary, and tertiary levels. Shortly after, it introduced DRG-based payments followed by global budgeting, both aimed at curbing supply-side moral hazard. However, the IT systems of the two clusters continued to go their separate ways, and it was only in 2004, under intense pressure from the Ministry of Health, that the two clusters finally accepted the creation of an electronic medical exhange that enabled sharing of medical records. There is no evidence that the splitting of Singapore's public health care institutions into two clusters has resulted in the healthy competition that would justify the increased overheads of maintaining two clusters, or that the health care providers, competing on price and quality, are rendering health care at the optimal point where marginal benefits justify the marginal costs. However, the realization that medical practice should be evidence-based rather than activity-based has recently led to the establishment of Health Services Research units at both clusters.

The Forces Fueling Change

It is pertinent to point out that shortly after coming into power in 1959, the PAP took an ideological right turn in the early 1960s, leading to its eventual withdrawal (or perhaps expulsion) from the Socialist International in 1976. Those were tumultuous years characterized by worker strikes and racial riots. With 30% of the popular vote left-leaning and the majority of the Chinese immigrant population emotionally attached to China and ideologically attuned to Chairman Mao's propaganda targeted at the Chinese Diaspora, there was fear that Singapore could well become the Cuba of Southeast Asia. As it turned out, the right wing of the party trumped the political left (from which it had openly split) in the battle for the hearts and minds of the people. Since then, Singapore has eschewed, at least rhetorically, egalitarian welfarism in favor of market mechanisms to allocate finite resources. Pragmatism, not ideology, would henceforth be the guiding principle.

What explains the people's ready acceptance of the government's hard-nosed policies with such heavy emphasis on individual responsibility? Again, it is necessary to understand the socio-politico-economic context. Firstly, Singaporeans had started out as poor hungry migrants escaping from the poverty and oppression of their original homelands — mainly China, India, and the Malay Archipelago. Despite 144 years of British colonial rule, the people did not benefit from a comprehensive NHS-style system of health care. Actually, British interest in the health of the locals was no different from that displayed by the Belgians in Africa, or the French in Indochina, or the Dutch in Indonesia: Western medicine on the heels of Western expansionism was principally concerned with the colonizers rather than the colonized. Local residents principally sought care from private traditional healers. Despite rampant poverty, malnutrition, overcrowding, and disease, there was no hospital and virtually no organised medical care for the low-income public in Singapore before the first charity hospital (Tan Tock Seng Hospital) was built in 1844, with funds raised by Chinese community leaders. Thus, the spirit of self-help is deeply ingrained in the Singaporean psyche. There is no tradition of state largesse.

Secondly, Singapore faced a most uncertain future at its birth in 1965. It had not sought independence but was unceremoniously ejected after its two-year political union with Malaysia failed. Cut off from its most vital hinterland, survival became the number one issue. Against all odds, Singapore not only survived but went on to become one of world's most prosperous countries with a per capita income in 2008 of US$52,900 (in Purchasing Power Parity, see Appendix). It was during those "sink-or-swim" years post-independence that a strong bond was forged between the government and the people. The people placed their trust in a sagacious government, which, in turn, earned more trust as it delivered more and more on its promises.

The pragmatic government fundamentally re-examined the role of the state vis-à-vis social welfare and concluded that a welfare state based on heavy taxes was not viable, indeed ruinous. It resolved not to let an "entitlement culture" creep in to overburden public finances, while ensuring that at all times appropriate safety nets were in place. It is telling that barely six months into office in 1960, the newly elected PAP government introduced user fees for outpatient services for the first time. The government charged 50 cents per visit to a government outpatient clinic. It was a small but symbolic step, which in hindsight was a harbinger of things to come. Convinced that health care cost is inherently inflationary, and the demand for it inherently insatiable, the government adopted "shared responsibility" as its guiding philosophy when it unveiled its National Health Plan in 1983: government would subsidize healthcare to make it affordable, but Singaporeans able to do so must contribute their share, too. A compulsory medical savings scheme would provide the needed mechanism to mobilize private financial resources.

Pragmatic Singaporeans, grateful for a standard of living previously only dreamed of, understood that trade-offs were an inevitable fact of life. They understood that whether the burden fell on taxes, Medisave, employer benefits, or insurance, it was ultimately Singaporeans them- selves who must pay — since taxes are paid by taxpayers, insurance premiums are paid by the insured, and employee medical benefits form part of wage costs. They also understood that overburdening the state or employers would affect the competitiveness of Singapore's externally ori- ented economy and ultimately, their own livelihoods. It, was, therefore, not difficult to convince the people that free health care in the face of potentially insatiable demand was illusory and potentially ruinous. Neither was it beyond them to grasp that the opposite extreme — fee-for- service open-ended insurance-based health care, which only the rich can afford — would be too inequitable. Hence, it was almost inevitable that a "third way" was found — but it was a path guided more by conscious avoidance of failed international models, than by a clear vision of what the perfect model might look like.

Search for Value and Efficiency through Competition

Having decided on how to finance health care, health reformers turned to achieving efficiency in its provision, in other words, getting value for the money spent. Although it had earlier failed in its attempt to privatize the public hospitals, the government firmly held on to its belief that compet- itive health care markets, in which public and private providers freely compete, would result in improved productivity, access, and quality — ultimately benefiting health care consumers.

An important element of market competition is consumer informa- tion. In 2003, the Ministry of Health mandated all hospitals in Singapore, both public and private, to declare the median size of their bills charged to patients. The bills include ward charges, doctors' professional fees, and all ancillary charges. Since then, the costs of 70 common medical procedures are published on the Ministry of Health's website and updated online on a monthly basis. With greater transparency of hospital bills, hospitals are now less indifferent towards cost to patients, and patients are now less ignorant of the comparative prices for the same medical treatment or procedure. CEOs of hospitals shown to have higher charges than others for the same treatment or procedure have had to scramble to either justify or slash fees. The starkest revision seen so far is for Lasik surgery, a procedure which surgically corrects short-sightedness. The price has dropped by about SG$1000 (US$708), or 40%, within 10 months at two leading institutions. The Singapore National Eye Centre, the most expensive center in 2003 (topping even the rates at the private sector's up-market facility in Mount Elizabeth Hospital), has since become the cheapest, raising questions from the public as to why such high prices had been allowed at all and for so long. Stroke treatment at Class B1 wards at the National University Hospital fell from SG$3141 (US$2223) to SG$2459 (US$1740). Private hospitals have since been included in the exercise. It was found that they had been charging between 20–120% more than the public hospitals for the same conditions listed.

Next, the Ministry of Health's website published comparative information on the bed situation and cost for intermediate and long-term care (ILTC) residential facilities. The list is updated at regular intervals. The aim is to allow Singaporeans to make more informed choices and provide the ILTC industry with comparative benchmarks and clearer market signals.

The Ministry of Health is also encouraging public-sector hospitals to outsource routine medical work so as to free up limited and expensive manpower who can then concentrate on higher-end value-added work. The successful introduction of teleradiology in Singapore, over the protests of local radiologists, illustrates this point. Teleradiology has been widely used in Singapore since 2005, and involves electronically tramsmitting X-rays from Singapore to Bangalore, India for processing. Reports come back within 30 minutes. The benefits for patients are enormous: instead of waiting two weeks to receive their X-ray results, patients now receive their results on the same day. Teleradiology also saves patients a second trip to the doctor, a second consultation fee, and a day's productivity at work. The Health Ministry had apparently done its work to garner support for the move: the presidents of the College of Radiologists, the Academy of Medicine of Singapore, and the Singapore Radiological Society publicly stated their support for "any initiative which could improve health care for patients," adding that they were specifically committed to ensuring that any radiology service provided to patients in Singapore, whether local or outsourced, is of the highest standard and cost-effective. The Ministry of Health, for its part, carries out randomized, double-blind quality control tests on the radiological readings, regardless of whether they are performed in Singapore or overseas. It argues that this is the best way to ensure that Singapore patients receive quality care that measures up to international benchmarks.

Quality and Patient Safety

Competition based on pricing, without reference to quality and patient safety, is meaningless. Singapore's journey in quality health care and patient safety has been discussed elsewhere (see Lim, 2004b). Suffice it to say, all hospitals have their own in-house quality assurance programs while the Ministry of Health centrally monitors their clinical performance. The goal is to create a culture of continuous quality improvement, safety consciousness, and public accountability. To ensure quality of care and patient safety, each hospital or specialist medical institution has a (mandated) Quality Steering Committee chaired by either the CEO or COO, which oversees all quality-related initiatives and monitors key performance indicators in the hospital. Regular meetings are devoted to customer satisfaction and business process reengineering, while hospital culture empowers staff to improve service standards and to reach "world-class" standards of service quality. More recently, in the last six to seven years, the focus has widened to include clinical quality and patient safety as well. While initially focused on "structural" approaches such as credentialing and accreditation, these efforts have come to include systematic measures of clinical processes and outcomes, as opposed to simply letting individual doctors decide what works best for their patients. Teams of quality managers have been engaged to monitor clinical quality indicators at the acute-care hospitals and benchmark them against national and international standards.

A new paradigm of health care regulation involving the participation of empowered consumers is emerging. The convergence of electronic medical records and case mix enables detailed tracking of the otherwise opaque clinical care processes, thus facilitating objective analysis of patient outcomes. At the Health Ministry's prodding, hospitals are now publishing selected quality indicators on their websites. Following the 2000 publication of the Institute of Medicine's landmark report, *To Err is Human*, and in light of growing awareness of medical errors and patient safety issues around the globe, the Ministry of Health recently expanded the duties of the Health Regulation Division (previously the Medical Audit and Accreditation Unit) to include risk management at the hospital level. The Health Regulation Division is already responsible for licensing and accreditation, legislative enforcement, surveillance, clinical audit, and quality assurance programs. Whereas the traditional approach had been to rely on Committees of Inquiries after the occurrence of an adverse event occurred, the new focus is on proactively preventing system failures through the reporting of "near-misses" (supplementing the existing critical incident reporting system) so that vulnerabilities in the system that may cause medical errors may be identified early on and rectified.

Changing Medical Practice: Disease Management Paradigm

Perhaps the most promising reform in health care provision undertaken thus far is the Ministry of Health's concerted effort to change the way medicine is practised in Singapore through its nation-wide "disease management" program, started in 2006. There is growing medical consensus worldwide that a holistic approach to chronic diseases can achieve better health outcomes while cutting costs. For example, if a diabetic patient works in close cooperation with doctors and nurses to achieve control over his or her blood sugar, serious and costly complications like blindness, kidney failure, or amputation can be avoided. The Ministry of Health has identified four chronic diseases for which there are established disease management (or clinical pathways) protocols: diabetes mellitus, hypertension, hyperlipidemia, and stroke. The program affects about one million Singaporeans, or one quarter of the total population and its success depends on patients' compliance and doctors' adherence to clinical practice guidelines. The Ministry of Health thus recruits private general practitioners (GPs) to sign up with the chronic disease management program, and hospital specialists discharge their patients with chronic illnesses to these receiving GPs. The latter track the patients' progress while simultaneously participating in hospital-run continuing medical education programs that keep GPs updated on the latest developments in chronic disease management.

The aim is also to progressively steer patients with chronic diseases, mainly by official encouragement and facilitation, towards a model of "seamless" care. This program is actually part of a larger public-private partnering initiative to encourage GPs to take care of patients who are in stable condition, thus substantially reducing the burden on overcrowded public hospitals. The Health Ministry therefore mounted a parallel campaign to inform the public that GPs are just as capable as specialists and, in fact, less expensive. The public has been assured that the GPs they see are actively upgrading their professional skills. Meanwhile, the GPs have the chance to demonstrate to the public that patients with chronic illnesses who require monitoring receive better and more responsive services if seen by a regular family physician instead of a hospital-based specialist.

To provide the right financial incentives for shifting the care of stable chronic conditions to primary care doctors, the Medisave purse strings were loosened in 2007 to allow patients with the four chronic conditions to use up to SG$300 (US$212) a year from Medisave to co-pay for their treatment. After one year of implementation, some 70,500 patients have withdrawn a total of SG$15 million (US$10.6 million) to pay for their outpatient treatment. Patients not only welcomed the financial relief of using Medisave money to cover the costs of consultations, but also reported traveling shorter distances to see their general practitioners and their relationship with their doctors improved as well.

But using the completion of regular examinations and tests prescribed by clinical protocols as a benchmark, the program exhibited room for improvement. Only 19% of diabetic patients had all the necessary tests done, while only 27% of patients who had suffered a stroke received a risk assessment for thromboembolism. About 62% of hypertensive patients and 77% of patients with high cholesterol got all the required checks. Of the diabetic patients with lipid disorders, nearly 50% fell within the ideal range of bad cholesterol level. But overall, about 70% of diabetic patients exhibited acceptable or better control of the disease.

Encouraged by the initial success of the Medisave for Chronic Disease Management Program, the government decided to include two more conditions in 2008: asthma and chronic obstructive pulmonary disease. It hopes that more of the patient load for chronic diseases can be shifted to general practitioners.

Conclusion

Singapore's health care system reflects a mix of strong market orientation and individualism, with a high acceptance level of government intervention. The combination of individual savings accounts with employer subsidies and public (means-tested) subsidies targeted at low-income families make for a quasi-private system under tight government control. The absence of a tradition of well-organized stakeholders and opposition groups has contributed to the rapid adoption of top-down policies. Patients are accustomed to cost sharing rather than depending on state largesse, but government subsidies keep basic health care affordable to most. The cost-sharing formula has to some extent countered the "moral hazard" generally associated with fee-for-service third party reimbursement. Recognizing the imperfections of the health care market, the government intervenes whenever it deems necessary. It tweaks incentives to encourage demand-side responsibility or discourage supply-side waste, in addition to generating competitive pressures for providers to be efficient.

Compared to the Organization for Economic Cooperation and Development (OECD) countries, Singapore has been very successful in containing the level of health care spending to below 4% of GDP. The government share of national health expenditure has steadily declined from 50% in 1965 to 21% in 2005. With first-world standards of health attainment — an average life expectancy of 80.6 years and an infant mortality rate of 2.1 per 1000 live births (Ministry of Health, 2007) — at an affordable 3–4% of GDP, Singaporeans appear to be getting good value for their money. It remains to be seen, however, whether this low level of spending can be maintained as Singapore's economy matures and economic growth inevitably slows down, lessening the masking effect of the expanding GDP denominator. (Lim, 2005).

Paradoxically, just as governments elsewhere are mulling over cutbacks in health spending, Singapore's health care planners are busy laying down the groundwork for the expansion and upgrading of its health facilities over the next 10 years — a move which will cost billions of dollars. There are two reasons for this. Firstly, their estimates show that the population needs to grow by another 2 million and stabilize at 6.5 million in order to generate the human capital needed to sustain Singapore's dynamic economy. This will have to be achieved largely through immigration, since natural births are woefully inadequate. Secondly, the government has committed to restructuring Singapore's economy and the Economic Review Committee (2002) has identified the Health Sector as an important target for economic growth. The government has, in fact, set a target of 1 million foreign patients by 2012, reckoning that it will generate SG$3 billion (US$2 billion) in revenue and create 13,000 new jobs in the process. Hence, demand for quality health care services, on both domestic and foreign fronts, cannot but rise. For Singapore's pragmatic government with a knack for turning necessity into virtue, this is not necessarily a bad thing.

References

Choo V. (2002). "Southeast Asian countries vie with each other to woo foreign patients." *The Lancet* **360**(9338): 1004.

Hsiao WC. (1995). "Medical savings accounts in Singapore." *Health Affairs* **14**(2): 260–266.

Lim MK. (1998). "Health care systems in transition II. Singapore, Part I. An overview of the health care system in Singapore." *J Public Health Med* **20**(1): 16–22.

Lim MK. (2004a). "Shifting the burden of health care finance: A case study of public-private partnership in Singapore." *Health Policy* **69**(1): 83–92.

Lim MK. (2004b). "Quest for quality care and patient safety: The case of Singapore." *Quality Safety Health Care* **13**(1): 71–75.

Lim MK. (2005). "Transforming Singapore health care: Public-private partnership." *Ann Acad Med Singapore* **34**(7): 461–467.

Ministry of Health. (2009). "Ministry of Health, Singapore." Accessed 4 March 2009. http://www.moh.gov.sg.

Phua KH. (1991). "Privatization and restructuring of health services in Singapore." *Institute of Policy Studies. Occasional Paper No. 5.* Time Academic Press, Singapore.

Preker AS, Harding A. (2003). *Innovations in Health Service Delivery: The Corporatization of Public Hospitals.* World Bank Publications, Washington, DC.

"Singapore Medicine, Singapore — A Global Affair." (2007). *Newsweek*, 5 October.

Yong YL. (1967). Speech by the Minister of Health at the Opening of the WHO Seminar on Health Planning in Urban Development. Singapore, 21 November.

Chapter 5

Consumer-Driven Versus Regulated Health Insurance in Switzerland

Luca Crivelli[*,†] *and Iva Bolgiani*[‡]

Introduction

In the last few years, the Swiss health system has been the object of particular attention in the United States (Leu *et al.*, 2009; Harris, 2007). In two articles published in the same issue of the *Journal of the American Medical Association*, Herzlinger and Parsi (2004) on the one hand and Reinhardt (2004) on the other outlined the main characteristics of the Swiss health insurance model. Both articles pointed out important lessons for the U.S., but while considering the same factuality, they proposed radically different hypotheses and explanations for the (alleged) superiority of the Swiss health care sector compared with that of the U.S. Ultimately, these authors drew very different conclusions.

While Swiss health care is based mainly on liberalism and private initiative, with ample freedom of choice for the patient-insured, it is heavily regulated by the state. Switzerland guarantees its citizens universal cover for a wide package of health care services with superior health outcomes and less pronounced inequalities than the U.S., but with a significantly lower percentage of GDP and per capita expense devoted to the health care sector (for an exhaustive review of the Swiss health system see: OECD, 2006). Both articles recognized that in Switzerland, the health care market

* Corresponding author.
† Università della Svizzera italiana and SUPSI. Email: Luca.Crivelli@usi.ch.
‡ University of Geneva.

is anything but free and perfectly functioning, since health insurance is compulsory, premiums and benefits are tightly controlled, "demand is constrained by mandated benefits, supply by uniform prices, and information about quality of providers is nonexistent" (Herzlinger and Parsi, 2004). However, Herzlinger and Parsi attributed Switzerland's superior economic performance to the fact that citizens in this country have adequate information about their insurers and thus health insurance is, at least partially, consumer-driven. In effect, Swiss citizens (and not employers or the government) buy health insurance plans, pay the bulk of health care expenses through insurance premiums, copayments, and out-of-pocket expenses, and choose the size of the deductible and other characteristics of the plan according to their own needs and preferences. In the opinion of Herzlinger and Parsi, the high cost transparency and the significant role of consumers in health care payments explain effective cost control as citizens can obtain what they consider "good value for their money." The interpretation offered by Reinhardt was diametrically opposite; he argued that the performance of the Swiss system must be ascribed to the pervasive government regulation and not to higher out-of-pocket costs borne by Swiss households or to the role of consumer choice. The insured in Switzerland have slight influence over the prices paid to providers, their choice is confined to a trade-off between cost sharing and premium rebate for the mandated benefit package, while the Swiss market for compulsory health insurance is dominated by considerable inertia, reflected in the high variance of premiums within cantons for the same insurance coverage.

It is difficult to establish which of the two interpretations comes closer to reality. Unfortunately, both articles yield to the temptation to stress the analogies between the Swiss and the American system, and in so doing underestimate the importance of the particular political and social context present in Switzerland.[1] In our opinion, it is not possible to

[1] For Reinhardt, the Swiss model substantially recalls the approach of the Clinton Health security plan: "It is not far-fetched to see in the Swiss health system a close cousin of the Clinton health security plan although it is, of course, not an identical twin" (p. 1230); for Herzlinger and Parsi, Switzerland includes some of the characteristics of the consumer-driven health care model, which some American economists would like to see as the future health care structure in the U.S.

understand the Swiss health system without paying attention to the role played by federalism and direct democracy on the one hand, and to the country's economic and social traditions on the other. These factors obviously play a major role in the current efforts to reform the Federal Health Insurance Law. This chapter aims to fill this gap in understanding, and illustrate how the institutions of federalism and direct democracy in Switzerland weaken both the role of the health insurer and the regulatory role of the state.

The first part of the chapter outlines the central role of individual sovereignty (through "voice" and "exit") in Swiss health care, focusing on the threefold role of citizen, insured, and patient (for a general reflection on exit, voice, and loyalty in the health care sector see: Klein, 1980). The second part evaluates the performance of the Swiss system from the point of view of both exit and voice mechanisms, and the final section focuses on the debate over health insurance reforms presently under consideration in Parliament. This final section outlines the tensions caused by the particular institutional features of the Swiss political system mentioned above, and presents two potential, radically different escape routes from the present situation.

The Governance of the Swiss Health System: Playing the Threefold Role of Citizen, Insured, and Patient by Using the Exit or Voice Option

The organization of the Swiss health system reflects at least three fundamental factors: a strongly decentralized political system based on federalism and the institutions of direct democracy, a liberal economic culture, and a well-developed tradition of social security. In the second half of the 20th century, the latter gave rise to universal social insurances (pensions, annuities for widows and orphans, disability insurance, unemployment insurance, family allowances) and state regulation in certain economic sectors, such as medical care (Achtermann and Berset, 2006). The Swiss political arena provides an intriguing case of particular arrangements for citizens' use of "exit" and "voice" to express their dissatisfaction and to force managers and politicians to adjust.

These core elements of the Swiss political system have shaped the relative weight assigned to the three roles that individuals usually play in health care: the roles of citizen, insured, and patient.[2] Switzerland (see Fig. 1) places strong emphasis on the idea that individuals should be able to exercise their "sovereignty" as citizens–voters as insured and as patients. The system therefore offers radical forms of voice and exit side by side. Voice is embedded in the institution of direct democracy, while exit strategies include the freedom to change health insurer every year,

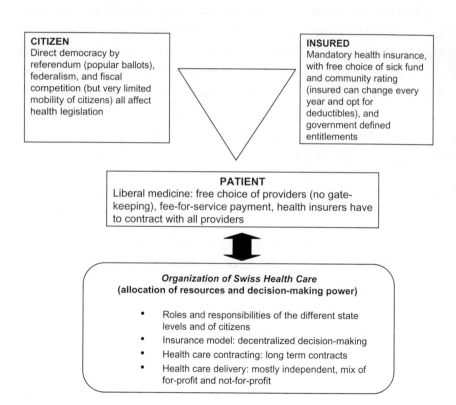

Fig. 1. The interplay of the roles of citizens, insured, and patients and the allocation of decision-making authority in Swiss health care.

[2] It is obvious that in universal health systems financed by means of taxations (Beveridge model), the role of the insured is less evident or is limited to private insurance contracts; on the other hand, the insured's role seems more central in Bismarckian systems and in health care markets based on consumers' free choice.

free choice of provider, and "liberal medicine" or professional autonomy. But as Hirschman (1970) already realized, the opportunity to resort simultaneously to these two reaction mechanisms can cause problems. The fact that individuals can choose between exit and voice has caused strong tensions in Switzerland. It also has contributed to weak governance of the Swiss health care system and to the profound crisis that has faced health insurance in recent years.

This chapter focuses on the tensions between voice in Switzerland's federal political sphere (by means of direct democracy) and the exit option in health insurance. In the last 10 years, the option to change insurer or insurance plan, inspired by liberal economic principles, has gained weight as a governance instrument in the health care sector (Swiss patients have had free choice of provider for many decades).

Voice in a Small Federal State with a Strong Tradition of Direct Democracy

Switzerland is a small federal state of 7.6 million inhabitants in the middle of Europe. It has 26 cantons, or provinces. Article 3 of the Swiss Constitution grants a high degree of autonomy to the cantons: "The cantons are sovereign insofar as their sovereignty is not limited by the Federal Constitution; they shall exercise all rights which are not transferred to the Confederation." The precept of the Swiss decentralization is that public policies and their implementation should be the responsibility of the lowest level of government capable of achieving the objectives (a notion somewhat similar to that of the "subsidiarity" of European Union politics). The cantons are thus responsible for health care regulation and supply as well as for the implementation of the federal health insurance law.

This decentralization of competences, combined with ample autonomy of the cantonal governments in public expenditure decisions[3] and fiscal federalism, has led to significant regional differences in levels of

---

[3] Public health expenditure (26% of total health expenditure) is predominantly provided for by cantons and municipalities.

health care expenditure and the dimension of production capacity (Crivelli, Filippini and Mosca, 2006). The differences between cantons extend to regulatory settings and the role of the private versus the public sector. Instead of a single health system, Switzerland's health care consists of 26 subsystems, connected to each other by the 1996 Federal Health Insurance Law (FHIL).

In a federal state, the citizen has the option to show his/her own preferences not only by means of the system of democratic representation, but also through the exit option, by "picking that community which best satisfies his preference pattern for public goods" (Tiebout, 1956), i.e. by voting with feet. Inman and Rubinfeld (2000) added: "The world of decentralized, competitive governments will allow for a national regulatory marketplace, in which individuals move among local jurisdictions or states to select the regulatory combination that they most desire." In such a context, "the pressure of taxpayers shopping, through exit and relocation, [will] force governments to be efficient in their provision of public goods and services." However, unlike the U.S., where citizens show great ("coast-to-coast") mobility, the exit option hardly plays a role in the Swiss political field. Although personal tax rates in Switzerland are more important for the location of business than corporate tax rates (Feld and Kirchgässner, 2003), since they are crucial for the attraction of highly skilled employees, the transfer from one canton to another is not viable for the majority of Swiss citizens due to the existing cultural and linguistic barriers between the regions. In the last few years, fiscal competition among cantons (especially regarding the taxation of mobile production factors) has been substantially augmented (Feld and Reulier, 2009). However, in the particular context of Switzerland, voice (by means of direct democracy) still plays the most relevant role. In the absence of an exit culture, the Swiss political system has facilitated the recourse to voice when citizens feel that political decisions do not adequately reflect their preferences; meanwhile, direct democracy has proven to cause significantly lower expenditure and revenue (Feld and Kirchgässner, 2005).

In fact, at both the cantonal and the federal level, citizens can participate directly in every state decision by means of direct democracy.

For example, federal laws and generally binding decisions of the Confederation are subject to an optional referendum. Such a referendum takes place when 50,000 citizens so request, and they must submit their signatures within 100 days of publication of a decree. The referendum is similar to a veto. It has the effect of delaying or blocking government policies or amendments adopted by Parliament. Commentators regularly label the referendum a "brake" on the political process, applied by the people.

A second way for citizens to induce policy change in the route is called the "popular initiative." If citizens want to propose a constitutional amendment and collect at least 100,000 signatures within 18 months of the initiative's launch, a popular ballot must be held. The outcome will be binding, provided that a majority of voters and of cantons support the proposal.

The combination of these two factors (direct democracy and federalism) has made the federal state particularly vulnerable. It greatly reduces the autonomy of both the central government and the federal administration, and has created a particularly decentralized and complex political system.

The Swiss health system is also based on these two institutional pillars. This had made the adoption of every legislative reform particularly difficult and slow. Direct democracy allows the Swiss citizen to intervene directly in decision-making (by approving or rejecting every reform in a popular ballot), while federalist arrangements encourage the proliferation of widely divergent organizational models and spending levels. In principle those differences reflect the preferences of the residents of the 26 cantons, but in practice they create inevitable tensions, and raise the question whether Switzerland will be able to maintain a universal insurance system at the national level.

Exit in a Mandatory Health Insurance System with Regulated Benefit Basket and Community-Rated Premiums

The Swiss health insurance system reflects features of both private and social insurance. On the one hand, the state plays a significant role in terms of regulation. For example, health insurance is mandatory for all residents, and it covers a package of health care benefits defined by law.[4] Premiums are community-rated by age group (under 18 years, 19–25 years, and older than 25 years) and by region, and subject to state regulation. People with low incomes can receive a state subsidy to help pay their health insurance premiums. At the same time, the health insurance has some elements of the private sector, since individuals are required to purchase their own basic health insurance by choosing from one of about 90 competing private insurance companies (nonprofit sick funds) that offer the basic insurance plan.[5] Moreover, since 1996, sick funds have been able to offer complementary health insurance on a for-profit base (which falls under private law).

In passing the 1996 Law on Health Insurance, the Swiss legislature drew its inspiration from the model of "managed competition,"[6] which had already been adopted or discussed by other European countries, including The Netherlands (Bolgiani *et al.*, 2006). This model is based on the premise that the rules of the free market do not work adequately in the health care sector[7]; consequently, an alternative approach to fostering competition in the system involves "shifting" the competition mechanism away from the direct relationship between patients and their physician to the relationship between health insurer and insured as well as the relationship between health insurer and health care provider. All citizens have to take out health insurance and

---

[4] It is important to point out that, until the FHIL came into force in 1996, health insurance was voluntary at the federal level. In 6 cantons, affiliation to a health insurance company was made compulsory for the whole population before 1994, and in 12 cantons, for special social groups (people with low income, and foreigners) — see Alber and Bernardi-Schenkluhn (1992).

[5] As in The Netherlands, the mandated health insurance of Switzerland raises the following question: To what extent should the insurance scheme be considered public or private? From the administrative perspective, it is a private scheme. Competing private insurance agencies are responsible for the administration. However, the scheme also has features of social insurance: mandatory subscription, community rating of premiums, with fiscal subsidy for low-income families. See also footnote 8 of the chapter on The Netherlands.

[6] This concept defines the mechanism of restricted competitive regulation proposed for the first time by Enthoven (1993, 2003). See also Enthoven (2005).

[7] For problems linked to the asymmetry of information, demand is not capable in any adequate manner of "managing" supply, which in fact enjoys considerable discretionary power. See Maynard (2005a, 2005b).

can freely choose an insurer, leaving it to the latter to exert competitive pressure on doctors and hospitals by negotiating contracts with providers and developing managed care arrangements and cost control mechanisms.

To enforce the "managed competition," the 1996 law strengthened the role of the exit mechanism as it made switching from one health insurer to another even easier than it had already been in the past.[8] The establishment of a uniform health insurance contract at the national level was one of the major reform elements of 1996. This standardization of the basic coverage aimed to guarantee the same benefit basket to all residents of Switzerland and to easily facilitate switching.[9] The FHIL established the same minimum amount of financial risk to be borne by the insured in the form of a mandatory annual deductible (totaling $180 PPP since 2004)[10] plus, for the yearly expenditure exceeding that deductible, a 10% copayment, up to a maximum amount of $420 PPP per year. Further, the law safeguarded universal access to all providers, as it required all health insurers to contract with all hospitals and physicians operating in the market (also known as mandatory contracting).

As a consequence, the basic health insurance offered by the different sick funds is the same for all, such that competition between health insurers should reflect only the quality of administrative services (time to reimburse bills, client support, etc.) and the premium (the flat-rate premium established by each insurer).[11] In order to facilitate switching

---

[8] Switzerland had substantial past experience with switching, primarily among low-risk individuals (Laske-Aldershof *et al.*, 2004).

[9] Since the benefit basket is established by federal law, no differences can exist in the coverage offered by the different competing sick funds or for people living in different cantons.

[10] PPP: 2007 purchasing power parity in US dollars ($1 = CHF 1.67).

[11] Although tie-in practices are forbidden, the ambivalent character of contractual relations between the health insurers (who offer, alongside basic insurance, private complementary cover in a less regulated market) raises serious difficulties for the insured in understanding the distinction between the two types of contract. If, in the mind of insured people, the two types of contract cannot be clearly separated, the contents of complementary insurance may influence the choice of basic insurance. More information on the relationship between basic and complementary cover in Swiss health insurance is provided in Crivelli (2009).

between sick funds, health insurers have to offer open enrollment; they have to accept anyone who requests basic coverage without setting restrictions for pre-existing conditions. Insured can change insurer twice a year (1 January and 1 July).[12]

Apart from this radical "full exit" (i.e. switching sick fund), the law includes two methods of "partial exit." The first option is for the insured to bear a higher amount of risk in exchange for a premium discount by selecting a higher deductible. The legislator sees this as an instrument to increase individual responsibility and to limit "moral hazard."

However, critics have pointed to the fact that there is empirical evidence that such premium discounts can lead to a process of adverse selection, as "good risks" (healthy and less costly insured) can partially escape the solidarity contribution toward bad risks implied by community rating.[13] In order to reduce risk selection, the law establishes a maximum deductible amount (of about $1500 PPP) and maximum premium discounts associated with different deductible levels.

The second option is for insurers to offer alternative insurance contracts (of the managed care type) that limit the freedom of patients to choose their provider. This has given rise to a variety of arrangements very similar to the U.S. Health Maintenance Organization (HMO), Preferred Provider Organizations (PPO), and Independent Practice Associations (IPA); in other words, networks of family doctors. The insured that sign up for such "managed care" contracts receive a premium discount. In theory, these alternative forms of insurance, whilst reimbursing the same range of services, should help to bring health care costs under control. Insurers can apply instruments such as selective contracting, gatekeeping, guidelines, and other management tools (e.g. case and disease management) to keep costs in check. The basic assumption of the 1996 reform was that over time the Swiss insured

---

[12] Some restrictions to change exist for special forms of insurance. For example, the insured persons who have chosen a higher deductible than the compulsory one may change sickness fund only once a year (1st January), and those who have opted for the "bonus-malus" model only every five years.

[13] See e.g. Geoffard *et al.* (2006).

would become more attentive and sensitive to such differences in plans and premiums (and therefore more mobile as well). An increase in the use of their "exit option" would encourage insurance companies to invest more in the aforementioned cost control instruments and reduce moral hazard.

Exit in the Swiss "Supermarket" of Medical Services

As mentioned above, the Swiss health system is based on a liberal conception of health and medicine. The patient–consumer's freedom of choice plays a central role. In this way, the Swiss health system resembles a huge health supermarket: patients freely shop around for the health care provider of their own choice, with excess capacity on the supply side. It is worth noting that Swiss patients have much wider access to diagnostic and therapeutic equipment than any other European nation. Further, Swiss physicians' incomes (in private surgeries, with the statute of free professionals) are higher than those of their colleagues in bordering countries (OECD, 2006).

The current law requires the sick funds to reimburse all medical services by physicians who have professional autonomy in determining the quality and volume of services. Mandatory contracting (the technical term for defining the present situation) ensures that all physicians who fulfill the requirements to practice have the right to sign a frame contract with all the health insurers.[14] By virtue of this obligation, patients are free to choose their own physician, can change their physician at any time, and are free to go directly to a specialist (there is no gatekeeping). This freedom of choice also applies to outpatient services that receive fee-for-service payment from the sick funds.

On the other hand, Swiss patients do not have access to full information about the clinical quality, efficacy, and appropriateness of the

---

[14] The only exception is represented by the insured who decide voluntarily, at least in part, to give up their right to the free choice of physician, and who opt for a special insurance form associated with managed care models in exchange for a reduction in the basic premium.

individual care providers; there is no public information about a physician's performance. Such information is indispensable if patients are to exercise conscious choices and enjoy real decisional autonomy. In fact, the exit option imagined by Hirschman presupposes the ability of consumers to react to poor quality of service by choosing other providers who perform better. In the Swiss health market, the chronic lack of information and transparency regarding the quality of health care (asymmetry of information between supply and demand) makes every reaction mechanism an illusion.

The federalist politics creates another obstacle to an effective exit option. In the small federal state with only seven million inhabitants, each of the 26 cantons is bound to plan the health care services for its own population by authorizing a sufficient number of health care facilities on its own territory or in the bordering cantons. The compulsory health insurance guarantees the reimbursement of hospital care for residents of each canton, and allows patients to seek hospital care in another canton in case of proven need. This provision encourages the creation of regional monopolies and segmentation of hospital supply that impedes the exploitation of potential economies of scale (Farsi and Filippini, 2006). It has also weakened competition between hospitals beyond regional borders.[15]

The Increasing Burden of Health Insurance Premiums as the Central Issue in Switzerland

In 2004, health costs in Switzerland overshot the psychological threshold of CHF 50 billion, or 11.6% of GDP (SFSO, 2006). With per capita health spending of $4055 PPP, Switzerland tops every other European country in terms of level and growth rate of health expenditure since the mid-1990s (SFSO, 2005). Overall, Swiss health care is characterized by substantial

---

[15] On the importance of promoting hospital competition beyond regional borders, see Porter and Teisberg (2006), and for an application to the Swiss hospital context, Teisberg (2008).

equity of access[16] and widespread satisfaction of the population, who feel that the system is very responsive to patients' preferences and offers ample freedom of choice.

However, the Swiss model's positive outcomes, mentioned in several recent international studies (WHO, 2000; Van Doorslaer *et al.*, 2002; OECD, 2006), are offset by its chronic inability to control health care expenditure and by the low level of technical efficiency (Zweifel, 2004). The explosion of health costs has translated into a continuous increase in health insurance premiums for the last 12 years. Between 1996 and 2008, the average per capita premium for adults increased by 82%, from CHF 2077 ($1243 PPP) to CHF 3775 ($2260 PPP), for annual cover.[17] This increase would have been even higher absent the shift of risks from health insurers to insured by means of a doubling of the minimum deductible (from CHF 150 to CHF 300, or $90 to $180 PPP), and absent the decision of the Federal Council to reduce the statutory reserve standards of insurers. So it is not surprising that the financial burden of health insurance premiums and user fees has become unsustainable for a large number of citizens (Bolgiani *et al.*, 2003). In fact, Switzerland has one of the most regressive health care financing systems in Europe (Wagstaff *et al.*, 1999).

Moreover, the situation is quite different from one canton to another. There is wide variation in premiums among the 26 cantons (see Fig. 2) and the Federal Constitution gives each cantonal authority the freedom to decide how much subsidy they can provide to families with modest incomes. To illustrate the degree of variation across cantons, we can quote

---

[16] Horizontal inequality scores for Switzerland are not significantly different from zero with respect to the probability of visiting a doctor and the mean number of visits, whereas the probability and number of GP visits are pro-poor and those of specialist visits are pro-rich (van Doorslaer, Masseria, and Koolman, 2006). However, according to some evidence on supply-induced demand in Switzerland (Crivelli *et al.*, 2006; Domenighetti *et al.*, 1993), we cannot exclude that in Switzerland the poor get the appropriate quantity of specialist visits while the rich show an overconsumption of specialist care.

[17] Great differences are recorded between one canton and the other. In percentages, the most important growth was noted in canton Thurgovia (+118%), and the lowest in Vaud (+45%). In absolute terms, the annual premium increased from a minimum of CHF 905 (in Nidwalden) to a maximum of CHF 2478 in Basle-Town (FOPH, 2006).

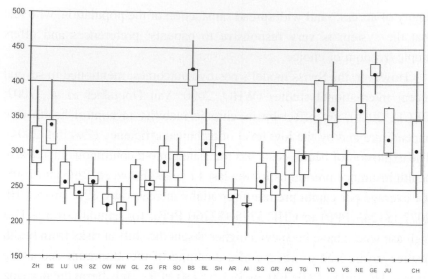

Source: Federal Office of Public Health, 2007.

Fig. 2. Monthly premium of compulsory health insurance: variations between insurers in 2008 (26 cantons and Switzerland as a whole).

the case of a family of four persons — two parents and two minor children — with a gross income of about $42,000 PPP. In 2007, this family would have paid 4.4% of their disposable income for health insurance if they resided in Canton Obwalden, whereas the burden would have been about 16.4% had they lived in Lausanne (Balthasar *et al.*, 2008).

Evaluation of the Resort to Exit

Over time the market structure of the health insurance industry has undergone profound change from a high number of small, local sick funds to a limited number of global players.[18] During this evolution mutual support

[18] Although there was an overall decrease in the number of insurers nationally, the average number of companies operating in each canton (i.e. the choice set from the insured's point of view) increased from an average of 40 funds per canton in 1997 to 56 in 2004 (Frank and Lamiraud, 2008). In 1980, the "global players" were just 1.8% of total sickness funds (Alber and Bernardi-Schenkluhn, 1992), while in 2008 the majority of health insurers (58%) are operating at the national scale.

groups were transformed into modern insurance companies, losing their local vocation and their link to particular population groups, such as employees in a given firm, members of a trade union, special professional categories, and inhabitants of a given area. Since 1996, the largest sick funds have increasingly lost clients, to the benefit of one insurance holding, which includes approximately 15 midsize sick funds and is adept at segmenting its clientele into risk groups. In the most recent years, even the largest sick funds have imitated this strategy, transforming themselves into holding companies, grouping sick funds that maintain their own company names but are managed according to a common strategic orientation.

Following Hirschman (1970), it is fair to assume that the power of the exit response is proportional to the elasticity of demand in response to quality deterioration. Therefore, an assessment of this reaction mechanism's functioning requires comprehensive data on health insurance switching related to variations in price and quality of the insurance cover. As explained above, for the standard contract there is no difference regarding the quality of the reimbursed medical care. Differences might exist, however, in the quality of the administrative services of insurers, and obviously in the community-rated premium they charge to their insured. The latter reflects, on the one hand, the average risk profile of the careers (thus sensitive to cream-skimming efforts of the insurer) and, on the other, the ability of the insurer to carry out an effective control of the invoices and to limit the consequences of moral hazard. There are tangible differences in the quality of the administrative service between one insurer and the other, but they are difficult to quantify.[19] It is even more difficult to determine the elasticity of demand with respect to administrative quality. What can be supposed is that these differences are more familiar to individuals who, for example as a result of a chronic illness, are obliged to communicate regularly with their insurers (as they would routinely require information or send invoices so that they can assess reimbursement celerity). For this reason, from a theoretical viewpoint, more competition among health insurers to acquire good risk and avoid

[19] See Comparis survey (www.comparis.ch).

bad risk could lead to a general decrease in the quality of client support services. It is thus hard to assess whether exit behavior creates an effective signal to the management of a given sick fund.

More information is available regarding the variation of premiums within the individual cantons. As shown in Fig. 2, there were substantial differences in premiums offered by the 40–70 health insurers operating within a given canton in 2008.

For example, in the canton of Zurich (ZH) in 2008, the monthly premium for the compulsory insurance for adults came to around CHF 265 ($159 PPP) with one of the least expensive insurers (5%-percentile), and to CHF 393 ($235 PPP) with one of the most expensive ones (95%-percentile), with an average amount around CHF 310 ($186 PPP). Despite the large differences in premiums (for an identical benefit basket) and despite the low costs of switching, only 2% of policyholders changed insurer between 2007 and 2008. This percentage (which is lower than that of the two previous years but in line with average movements of the last ten years[20]) includes movements between companies of the same insurance group.[21] According to Beck (2004), the price elasticity for mandatory health insurance estimated from aggregate (market share) data is around −0.5 in Switzerland, a value that is higher than in The Netherlands but much lower than in Germany (Schut *et al.*, 2003). Empirical evidence shows that the people willing to frequently change sick fund belong to the category of good risks (young, healthy, and higher-educated enrollees) (Beck *et al.*, 2003; Strombom *et al.*, 2002).

These data reveal that the majority of insured persons do not exit but stick with their insurance company even if premiums are 30–45% higher than the least expensive offer. According to Laske-Aldershof *et al.* (2004), the poor risk adjustment formula used in Switzerland, the favorable risk profile of the switchers, and the successful risk selection

---

[20] See Comparis survey (www.comparis.ch) and Colombo (2001).

[21] The three largest insurance groups operating in Switzerland (with a joint market share of 35%) established within themselves new health insurers that offer lower flat-rate premiums so as to attract good risks. Sometimes filling out a membership form has to be done via the Internet, which can be a barrier for elderly people (bad risks).

strategies adopted by sick funds have led to increased premium variation among Swiss funds over time.

There are two possible ways of interpreting this limited switching. On the one hand, the majority of insured may perceive the information and transaction costs of switching health insurers as very high.[22] On the other hand, this low mobility can be explained by loyalty. In fact, many insured people in Switzerland show a great degree of loyalty to their own sick fund, even while other funds may be cheaper. Many insured are risk-averse people, who prefer to remain faithful to a company whose faults and merits they know rather than face the uncertainty of a new insurer. Or perhaps, more simply, they remain confident that their own insurer will go back to offering the basic cover under competitive conditions after a few years. However, the opportunity for partial exit remains an option for people who do not wish to switch insurers: the choice of a higher deductible or a managed care contract.

As shown in Fig. 3, the number of adult insured who went for an optional deductible between 1997 and 2007 increased slightly. The largest increase is in the high band of deductibles (at least CHF 1200 per year, or $720 PPP), while the average levels of deductibles (between CHF 400 and CHF 1000 francs, or $240 and $600 PPP) clearly decreased.[23] Without doubt, the process of self-selection lies behind these changes. Geoffard *et al.* (2006) studied a representative sample of clients of a large sick fund. They found that the death rate of the insured who had selected the minimum deductible was 200% higher than that of those with an average deductible. On the other hand, the insured who had selected a high deductible had a 30% lower mortality rate than those

[22] A particular element might contribute to raising transaction costs. As indicated in the previous paragraph, health insurers may propose, alongside basic insurance, complementary insurance contracts, subject to private law. For these products, customer mobility is limited due to the fact that, when taking out such a policy, the insurer may request a medical examination and use the information obtained to calculate risk-adjusted premiums and to introduce limits to coverage in the contract. Some people fear that by changing the basic insurer they would lose the complementary cover.

[23] The maximum deductible went from CHF 1500 in 1996 to the present CHF 2500 francs.

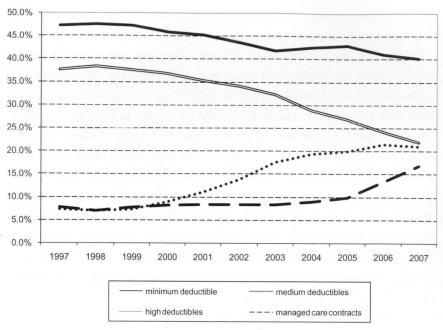

Source: Federal Office of Public Health, 2008.

Fig. 3. Percentage of the adult population having chosen minimum, medium, or high deductibles or managed care contracts.

with an average deductible, when the data were standardized by age and sex.

The exit of Swiss insured toward managed care contracts has been modest; in 2007, 16.9% of the adult population had opted for one of these alternative insurance forms.[24] After an initial burst of enthusiasm for managed care contracts in 1996, a period of stagnation ensued from 1997 to 2004, followed by an upsurge in the popularity of such contracts since

---

[24] It is important to note that there are sizeable differences in the spread of these special forms of insurance across cantons: in some cantons, 20–35% of the insured decided to limit freedom of choice with regard to the doctor, whereas in other cantons less than 5% of the population have decided to pursue alternative insurance. In particular, in the French- and Italian-speaking cantons, only a small number of people have opted for these alterative insurance models.

2005.[25] Indeed, instead of switching health insurers, a growing number of policyholders are opting for these alternative models to avoid premium increases for the "classic" form of insurance. Experts feel that the still modest spread of capitation-based managed care does little to enhance competitive pressure on health care providers; they argue that the plans do not offer enough discounts to overcome consumer resistance to managed care restrictions (Zweifel *et al.*, 2006). Lehmann and Zweifel (2004) compared the differences in (risk-adjusted) health costs between members of the three most widespread forms of managed care (HMO, PPO, IPA) and clients with traditional contracts. They found that patients with HMOs had 62% lower costs, those in PPOs 39% lower costs, and those in IPA 34% lower costs than the average. The law only allows insurers to offer a premium discount of 20%. After controlling for the effects of risk selection, the "true" savings account for two-thirds of the cost reductions recorded by HMOs, half of those by PPOs, and one-third of savings by IPAs. Since, especially in HMOs, clients only partially benefit from the savings in the form of a premium discount, it is quite probable that the people who signed up were in good health but making relatively little income and thus could not pay the full regular premium.

Evaluation of the Resort to Voice

Direct democracy and federalism are the main barriers to major and rapid reform in Swiss health care. The political system encourages marginal and incremental change (a step-by-step strategy). To anticipate the risk of veto, the government collects the opinion of the important interest groups on a given draft bill during the preparliamentary phase. As the bill enters the discussions in Parliament, it has already incorporated the claims of the most powerful actors, including professional associations, political parties, and movements that enjoy a reputation for winning majorities in referendum votes (Papadopoulos, 2001). In some cases, when Parliament cannot prevent recourse to direct democracy, it engages in *ex post*

---

[25] Between 1996 and 1997, membership in alternative insurance models quadrupled.

negotiations to explore whether it can meet the opponents' objections in a formal counterproject (a more moderate constitutional amendment) or, more frequently, in legislative amendments that do not require a popular vote. Moreover, unbalanced and radical revisions have a high likelihood of being rejected in popular ballots. The total revision of the Federal Health Insurance Law (FHIL) was approved in 1994 — a full 83 years after the law came into force in 1911, and after several years of debate, negotiation, and rejection of proposals in popular votes. Between 1974 and 2008, the Swiss population was called to the ballot box not less than 12 times to deliberate on health insurance reforms. The popular ballot rejected nine of those proposals (one proposal by Parliament, six popular initiatives, and two counterprojects) but accepted the referendum on the federal law in 1994 and two minor changes proposed in the form of an urgent federal decree (see Table 1).

The structural change of health care financing is a sound example of the obstacles to radical reform in Switzerland. In the last decade, there have been several attempts to improve the equity in financing by more adequate recourse to fiscal withdrawal[26] or by a change from community-rated premiums to income-dependent health insurance contributions.[27] The popular vote has rejected such radical change in the system four times and with a sweeping majority, between 60% and 70% (but each time with a participation rate of less than 50% of citizens, ranging from 39.7% in 1974 to 49.7% in 2003). The 2003 popular ballot provides an emblematic example. According to two surveys in 2002, a substantial majority of the Swiss (63%) declared themselves willing to pay health insurance contributions proportional to their income (Crivelli, Domenighetti and Filippini, 2006). However, six months later, in May 2003, 73% of voters rejected the popular initiative, "Health at Accessible Prices," which proposed a mixed financing system, including contributions dependent on income and on wealth, alongside an increase in TVA. Without doubt, there

[26] The popular initiative, voted on in 1992, suggested anchoring sufficient premium reductions in the Constitution, financed by the Confederation and cantons, to benefit people with modest income.
[27] With three popular ballots, in 1974, 1994, and 2003.

Table 1. History of Popular Ballots and Legislative Reforms in the Field of Federal Health Insurance

1900	Law Forrer rejected in referendum (by 70% of voters) Participation rate: 66.7%
1912	**Federal Law of Sickness and Accident Insurance (KUVG) accepted in referendum (by 54.5% of voters)** Participation rate: 64.3%
1964	**Partial revision of the KUVG** (the minor changes were accepted without popular ballot)
1974	Failure of a popular initiative (rejected by 70% of voting people and all cantons) and rejection of the counterproposal (by 61% of voting people and all cantons) Participation rate: 39.2%
1985	**Urgent federal decree accepted in referendum (by 53% of voters)** Participation rate: 34.7%
1987	Law amendment rejected in referendum (by 71% of voters) Participation rate: 47.6% Start of the preparatory work for the KVG
1992	Failure of a popular initiative (rejected by 60% of voting people and all but one of the cantons) Participation rate: 44.4%
1993	**Urgent federal decree accepted in referendum (by 80% of voters)** Participation rate: 39.8%
1994	Failure of a popular initiative (rejected by 76% of voting people and all cantons) and **the KVG accepted in referendum by 51.8% of voters** Participation rate: 43.8%
2000	Failure of a popular initiative (rejected by 82% of voting people and all cantons) Participation rate: 41.7%
2001	**1st revision of the KVG (no popular ballot requested)**
2003	Failure of a popular initiative (rejected by 73% of voting people and all cantons) Participation rate: 49.7% Failure in Parliament of the 2nd revision of the KVG
2004	Start in Parliament of a new approach to the 2nd revision of the KVG (unbundling strategy)
2007	Failure of a popular initiative (rejected by 72% of voting people and 21 cantons) Participation rate: 45.9%
2008	Failure of the referendum on the counterproject to the withdrawn popular initiative "for lower insurance premiums" (rejected by 69.5% of voting people and all cantons) Participation rate: 43.7%

were substantial differences between the (generic) question asked of the sample interviewed in the two surveys and the specific model proposed by the initiative's promoters. Moreover, the media campaign that began at the end of 2002 certainly persuaded many citizens that it was in their interest to maintain the status quo (see e.g. Credit Suisse, 2003).

Yet, in our opinion, there is a further explanation, which recalls Hirschman's theory. The opportunity for "exit" (to sick funds with lower premiums, higher deductibles, and managed care contracts) reduces the strength of "voice." Many people (especially those considered good risks and those with modest incomes) who in the absence of this "exit" opportunity would probably vote in favor of radical reforms of the system, end up not participating in popular ballots. When it is a question of voting on reforms in the health system, natural tensions occur within each individual, since the interests of the patient[28] diverge from those of the citizen and insured.[29] The low geographic mobility of the Swiss (which limits the chance to move to another canton — choosing exit as citizens) and the constraints on patients' mobility (whose chance to be treated in out-of-canton hospitals is subordinate to the canton's authorization) contrast sharply with the ample opportunities for exit that the present system offers the insured. In this way exit weakens voice, and in popular ballots there is less "protest" in support of the insured's interests.

There is a second institutional barrier to radical reforms: the distribution of responsibility and expenditure between cantons and the Confederation (Crivelli and Filippini, 2003). Although the Federal Constitution assigns the cantons sovereignty in the health care realm, the Confederation has played an increasingly active role in the health field since the introduction of the FHIL in 1996. Experts expect the Confederation to play an even more important role in defining the future of Swiss health policy as it aims to reduce regional differences in health care provision and economic burdens and implement cost control instruments at the national level

---

[28] Maintaining maximum freedom of choice when choosing a physician, not closing hospitals in the own region, keeping the bundle of insured services as adequate as possible.
[29] Paying fewer taxes respectively, avoiding continuous premium increases.

(Achtermann and Berset, 2006). However, the Confederation cannot take up these new tasks without an amendment to the Federal Constitution accompanied by an increase in public health expenditure on the federal level. In the absence of a constitutional change, the cantons, which today bear more than 90% of public health expenditure, are not willing to accept such radical expansion of the central state's (or health insurers') decision-making power without an equivalent transfer of financial responsibilities. So it is not surprising that the main opponents of the federal government's spring 2004 reform roadmap were the cantonal authorities themselves.

Finally, there is a third problem that brings changes of a cultural order into question. The obligation of Swiss citizens to insure themselves in conjunction with (radical and partial) forms of exit has altered their perception of what they are paying premiums for. As Oestrom (2000) has emphasized well, some policies may crowd out reciprocity and collective action. The impossibility of backing out of paying a premium (which, we mention again, is compulsory but independent of the ability to pay) has prompted many Swiss citizens to perceive health insurance as a socially unjust tax. At the same time, the possibility (and the invitation) to frequently change health insurer erodes the values of solidarity and mutuality typical of social insurances. In recent years, growing numbers of citizens have perceived covering against the risk of sickness as a commodity: they pay a premium in exchange for health care services (rather than transfer a financial risk to third parties in case illness strikes). The absence of any barriers for patients to access medical care and the "inflationist" incentives in the Swiss system encourage the consumption of unnecessary diagnostic and therapeutic services by people who are in good health (moral hazard *ex post*). The image of a welfare state in which "abuses are the order of the day" has spread through society, undermining the legitimacy of proposals aimed at maintaining or strengthening solidarity between the healthy and sick, young and old, rich and poor (Fong, Bowles and Gintis, 2005). This even threatens to undermine the very foundation of the universal insurance cover.

The Path of Health Insurance Changes: Reform or Revolution?

The previous sections discussed how the current law on Swiss health insurance represents a fragile compromise between market mechanisms and state regulation. The interaction between these two elements, as we have seen, hampers efficient governance of the system (Zweifel, 2004) and generates tensions between the three roles which individuals play in the health sector as citizen, insured, and patient. Opportunities for "voice" rest mainly with the citizens by means of direct democracy, while "exit" is in fact accessible only with regard to basic health insurance (given the lack of available information for patients to exercise effective choice).[30]

In the search for radical solutions to the problems outlined above, civil society has produced two starkly opposite popular initiatives. Despite the negative outcome of both popular ballots, in the near future the legislator and the Swiss people will be called on to make an important strategic decision — a decision that might break down the current fragile compromise between the elements of market and state regulation in health legislation.

Reforms Under the Banner of Continuity: The Swiss Government's Proposals

The government presented its reform proposals to the Federal Parliament in 2004; the ultimate objective of the proposals was to bring health expenditure under control (Swiss Federal Council, 2004). The enactment of the FHIL in 1996 has not greatly improved cost containment. This is mainly due to the ineffectiveness of instruments aimed at fostering competition in the health insurance market (free movement between health insurers, new insurance models of the managed care type, etc.) in a regulated and rather inflexible sector (including state-sponsored or state-controlled hospital planning, community-rated premiums, mandatory contracting with all

---

[30] And it will be in an even more marked way if the reforms presently under discussion are accepted.

160

service providers, compulsory benefit basket, and negotiation of fees). Furthermore, the complexity of the system and the diverging interests of the various actors (health care providers, insurers and other third-party payers, patients–insured–citizens) have made control over health expenditure more difficult.

After Parliament rejected a wide-ranging revision of the FHIL in 2003, the government decided to adopt a new approach in 2004. Although part of a uniform strategy (aimed at increasing competition and individual empowerment), the government presented its plan in a set of distinct legislative proposals so as to prevent the rejection of the entire package by Parliament, or, in the event of a referendum, by the Swiss people. The proposals focused especially on the demand side (Bolgiani *et al.*, 2006). They sought to encourage citizens to opt for alternative managed care plans, and also encouraged the creation of integrated networks of care with budget responsibility. Another goal was to heighten patients' awareness of health care costs by increasing deductibles and copayments. Further, substantial improvements in the risk adjustment formula would make risk selection less attractive to health insurers. The most controversial proposal sought to abandon mandatory contracting for insurers; the notion was that through selective contracting, quality of care would become a distinguishing factor in the selection of insurance plans. Changes in hospitals' funding mechanism would increase citizens' choice between public and private providers and increase competition between the two. Finally, the proposals reduced the collective funding for elderly care by eliminating some nursing and home care services from the mandatory basic coverage.

In spite of the declared objective, to achieve a system driven completely by market forces (in the future, Swiss insured will have a wider choice of insurance plans), the roadmap provided for step-by-step change, keeping a balance among the political forces of the country in order to avoid the brake of a popular ballot. If Parliament agrees with the proposals, the most likely outcome for the years to come will be hybrid solutions that will, once again, increase the tensions between the roles of citizen, insured, and patient while not really curbing the growth of expenditure.

Revolutions: The Proposals of a Part of Swiss Civil Society

Recently, the Swiss people rejected two fundamental system changes proposed by Swiss civil society in the form of two quite different initiatives. The first reform proposal aimed to strengthen the role of the state by setting up a single health insurer; the second aimed to strengthen the role of market and competition by minimizing state intervention and deregulation. Both sought to amend the present Federal Constitution and thus required the support of the majority of the people and cantons. The ballots took place in 2007 and 2008. The outcomes, once again, confirm the tensions present in a system that tries to reconcile state and market, sometimes in an extreme fashion. In fact, as in other countries, the left side of the political spectrum voices criticism of the failing results of competition among health insurers, and maintains that the inequitable financing of flat premiums is socially unsustainable. Right-wing political groups, in contrast, identify the problems of the Swiss health system as state constraints that prevent effective competition between sick funds, combined with excessive benefits that encourage overconsumption and moral hazard on the part of many patients. The Swiss population, facing the choice between these two radical alternatives (more state control and the resulting strengthening of voice, or more market control and the resulting strengthening of exit), opted by a large majority for maintenance of the status quo.

The modest results of competition among sick funds prompted the promoters of the 2007 initiative to propose a single insurer offering uniform entitlements for all Swiss citizens, with premiums dependent on the insured's ability to pay (Swiss Federal Council, 2005a). The Popular Movement for Families, sustained by the political left, was its main supporter. The initiative reflected fundamental principles of solidarity and efficiency by means of collective optimization of the insurance mechanism. It also aimed to increase the insurers' transparency and accountability, create a clear separation of compulsory and complementary insurance, and reduce administrative costs due to inefficiencies in the present system. The initiative clearly favored the voice mechanism, as it proposed ample citizen surveillance of the single health insurer, including the opportunity for the insured to be represented on the boards of directors. In fact, the exit option would have gradually disappeared, but enrollees would have gained more democratic power (voice), as they would have been able to intervene directly in the daily management of the health insurance.

The 2008 initiative, supported by the Swiss People's Party (a party on the right of the Swiss political spectrum), aimed to reduce the basic insurance premiums. Its two fundamental pillars were shifting part of the services from the compulsory benefit basket to complementary private insurances,[31] and strengthening exit in health insurance by means of market deregulation (e.g. abandoning mandatory contracting, liberalization of fees, and abandoning the mandatory contracting with all providers by the health insurers).[32] Parliament drew up a counterproject to this initiative called "For a More Effective and Better Quality Health Care System Thanks to Greater Competition." This proposal's objective was to anchor the most important principles of the initiative within the Federal Constitution, and to dismiss aspects (like the reduction of the benefit basket) with a very low probability of reaching a consensus. In January 2008, the Swiss People's Party decided to withdraw its initiative and to completely support this counterproject. If the constitutional change had passed, market mechanisms would have ruled relations between insurers and suppliers of care (e.g. selective contracting between insurers and suppliers, or insurers as single buyer due to the monistic financing of hospitals). The application of managed care instruments would have

---

[31] According to the proposals of the initiatives' promoters, the basic insurance should cover only the costs of medical treatments that serve to soothe pain, cure, and reintegrate the patient — treamtments that are adequate and economical and whose efficacy is recognized by science.

[32] We recall that at present the cantons cover at least 50% of the operative costs and 100% of the investments in public-interest hospitals by means of fiscal withdrawal. The promoters of the proposal suggested that this money should be transferred (in the form of a capitation fee) to the health insurers, who at this point would become the single buyers of all the insured health care services and would be held to cover the entire cost.

weakened the social insurance character of health insurance, but above all it would have transferred an important part of the decision-making power to insurers, to the detriment of politics and direct democracy. The fundamental consequence of ending mandatory contracting and entrusting the health insurer with the role of single buyer of all services is the restricted voice of citizens, who today have the right to express themselves on important topics such as hospital planning. The application of these new market elements would have eroded some pillars of the present legislation, in particular public determination of health coverage and the principle of solidarity.

As shown in Fig. 4, there is a clear cantonal divide in the popular support for the two ballots. Although both reform proposals were far from

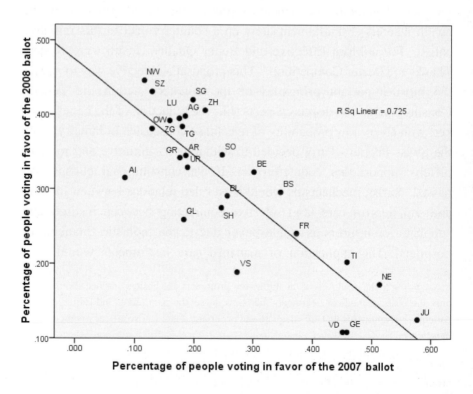

Fig. 4. Relationship among the cantonal results of the 2007 and 2008 ballots.

obtaining the needed dual majority (of the people and of the cantons) to pass, they pushed the debate on the reforms toward a well-defined strategic choice. It clarified not only the intended role of market mechanisms and state regulation, but also the dominant governance mechanism of Swiss health care: that of citizens, patients, or insured people. The reform proposals had the merit of bringing a series of elements into the public arena and the media that highlighted the limits of the present system and the need to better articulate the roles and functions of each actor in the system. The continuous pressure on costs and, as a result, on premiums makes a reorganization of the Swiss health system essential, and with it the search for a new equilibrium among freedom of choice, personal responsibility, pluralism, and the role of the state.

References

Alber J, Bernardi-Schenkluhn B. (1992). *Westeuropäische Gesundheitssysteme im Vergleich: Bundesrepublik Deutschland, Schweiz, Frankreich, Italien, Grossbritannien* ["Health Care Systems of Western Europe: Western Germany, Switzerland, France, Italy, and Great Britain"]. Campus, Frankfurt.

Achtermann W, Berset C. (2006). *Les Politiques Suisses De Santé — Potentiel Pour une Politique Nationale* ["Swiss Health Politics — Potential for National Policy-Making"]. Bern: Federal Office of Public Health.

Balthasar A, Bieri O, Gysin B. (2008). *Monitoring 2007. Die Sozialpolitische Wirksamkeit der Prämienverbilligung in den Kantonen* ["The Effectiveness of Earmarked Subsidies"]. Federal Office of Public Health.

Balthasar A, Bieri O, Müller F. (2005). *Monitoring 2004. Die Sozialpolitische Wirksamkeit der Prämienverbilligung in den Kantonen* ["The Effectiveness of Earmarked Subsidies"]. Federal Office of Public Health.

Beck K. (2004). *Risiko Krankenversicherung — Risikomanagement in Einem Regulierten Krankenversicherungsmarkt* ["Health Insurance Risks — Managing Risk in a Regulated Insurance Market"]. Bern: Paul Haupt Verlag.

Beck K, Spycher S, Holly A, Gardiol L. (2003). "Risk adjustment in Switzerland." *Health Policy* **65**(1): 63–74.

Bolgiani I, Domenighetti G, Quaglia J. (2003). "Satisfaction des Suisses à l'égard des Soins de Santé et des Primes de l'Assurance-Maladie" ["Satisfaction of the Swiss about health care and health insurance premiums"]. *Sécurité Sociale* **4**: 219–222.

Bolgiani I, Crivelli L, Domenighetti G. (2006). "The role of health insurance in regulating the Swiss health care system." *Revue Française des Affaires Sociales* **60**(3): 227–249.

Colombo F. (2001). *Towards More Choice in Social Protection? Individual Choice of Insurer in Basic Mandatory Health Insurance in Switzerland. Occasional Papers No. 53.* Organization for Economic Cooperation and Development, Paris. Accessed 23 February 2009. http://www.sourceoecd.org/10.1787/664178220717.

Credit Suisse. (2003). "Spotlight: Risques et effets secondaires de l'Initiative-santé du PS." Accessed 23 February 2009. https://marketdataresearch.creditsuisse.com/cs/mdr/p/d/qrr/research/files/getfiles.do?fileName=F071025000680.pdf.

Crivelli L. (2010). "Consumer driven health insurance in Switzerland, where politics are governed by Federalism and direct democracy." In: Thomson S, Mossialos E, Evans R (eds.), *Private Health Insurance and Medical Savings Accounts: Lessons from International Experience.* Cambridge University Press (forthcoming), Cambridge.

Crivelli L, Filippini M. (2003). "Il Federalismo nel Settore Sanitario ["Federalism in Health Care"]." In: Ghiringhelli A (ed.), *Il Ticino nella Svizzera* ["Ticino within Switzerland"]. Dadò, Locarno.

Crivelli L, Domenighetti G, Filippini M. (2006). "Federalism versus social citizenship: Investigating the preference for equity in health care." In: Bruni L, Porta PL (eds.), *Handbook on the Economics of Happiness.* Edward Elgar, Cheltenham.

Crivelli L, Filippini M, Mosca I. (2006). "Federalism and regional health care expenditures: An empirical analysis for the Swiss Cantons." *Health Econ Lett* **15**(5): 535–541.

Domenighetti G, Gutzwiller F, Martinoli S, Casabianca A. (1993). "Revisiting the most informed consumer of surgical service: The physician patient." *Int J Tech Assess Health Care* **9**(4): 505–513.

Enthoven A. (1993). "The history and principles of managed competition." *Health Affairs* **12**(Suppl): 24–48.

Enthoven A. (2003). "Employment-based health insurance is failing: Now what?" *Health Affairs* Web Exclusive, 28 May. Accessed 23 February 2009. www.healthaffairs.org.

Enthoven A, Tollen LA. (2005). "Competition in health care: It takes systems to pursue quality and efficiency." *Health Affairs* Web Exclusive, 7 September. Accessed 23 February 2009. www.healthaffairs.org.

Farsi M, Filippini M. (2006). "An analysis of efficiency and productivity in Swiss hospitals." *Swiss J Econ Stats* **142**(1): 1–37.

Feld LP, Reulier E. (2009). "Strategic tax competition in Switzerland: Evidence from a panel of the Swiss Cantons." *German Econ Rev* **10**(1): 91–114.

Feld LP, Kirchgässner G. (2003). "The impact of corporate and personal income taxes on the location of firms and on employment: Some panel evidence for the Swiss Cantons." *J Pub Econ* **87**(1): 129–155.

Feld LP, Kirchgässner G. (2005). "Sustainable fiscal policy in a federal system: Switzerland as an example." In: Kriesi H, Farago P, Kohli M, Zarin-Nejadan M (eds.), *Contemporary Switzerland: Revisiting the Special Case.* Palgrave MacMillan, Basingstoke:

Fong CM, Bowles S, Gintis H. (2005). "Reciprocity and the welfare state." In: Gintis H, Boyd S, Fehr E (eds.), *Moral Sentiments and Material Interests.* MIT Press, Cambridge.

FOPH. (2006). *Statistik der Obligatorischen Krankenversicherungen 2004* ["Social Health Insurance Statistics 2004"]. Federal Office of Public Health, Bern.

Frank R, Lamiraud K. (2008). "Choice, price competition and complexity in markets for health insurance." National Bureau of Economic Research, Working Paper No. 13817.

Geoffard PY, Gardiol L, Grandchamp C. (2006). "Separating selection and incentive effects: An econometric study of Swiss health insurance claims data." In: Chiappori PA, Gollier C (eds.), *Competitive Failures in Insurance Markets.* MIT Press, Cambridge.

Harris G. (2007). "Looking at the Dutch and Swiss health systems." *The New York Times*, 30 October.

Herzlinger RE, Parsa-Parsi R. (2004). "Consumer-driven health care." *J Am Med Assoc* **292**(10): 1213–1220.

Hirschman A. (1970). *Exit, Voice and Loyalty. Responses to Decline in Firms, Organizations, and States.* Harvard University Press, Cambridge.

Inman R, Rubinfeld DL. (2000). "Federalism." In: Bouckaert B, DeGeest G (eds.), *Encyclopedia of Law and Economics.* Edward Elgar, Cheltenham.

Klein R. (1980). "Models of man and models of policy: Reflections on exit, voice, and loyalty ten years later." *Milbank Mem Fund Quart: Health Soc* **58**(3): 416–429.

Laske-Aldershof T, Schut E, Beck K, Shmueli A, Van de Voorde C. (2004). "Consumer mobility in social health insurance markets: A five-country comparison." *Appl Health Econ Health Policy* **3**(4): 229–241.

Lehmann HJ, Zweifel P. (2004). "Innovation and risk selection in regulated social health insurance." *J Health Econ* **23**(12): 997–1012.

Leu RE, Rutten FH, Brouwer W, Matter P, Ruetschi C. (2009). *The Swiss and Dutch Health Insurance Systems: Universal Coverage and Regulated Competitive Markets.* The Commonwealth Fund, New York.

Maynard A. (2005a). "Common challenges in healthcare markets." In: Maynard A (ed.), *The Public–Private Mix for Health.* Radcliffe, Oxford.

Maynard A. (2005b). "Enduring problems in healthcare delivery." In: Maynard A (ed.), *The Public–Private Mix for Health.* Radcliffe, Oxford.

OECD. (2006). *Review of the Swiss Health System.* Paris: OECD.

Ostrom E. (2005). "Policies that crowd out reciprocity and collective action." In: Gintis H, Boyd S, Fehr E (eds.), *Moral Sentiments and Material Interests.* MIT Press, Cambridge.

Papadopoulos Y. (2001). "How does direct democracy matter? The impact of referendum votes on politics and policy-making." In: Lane JE (ed.), *The Swiss Labyrinth: Institutions, Outcomes and Redesign.* Frank Cass, London, Portland.

Porter ME, Teisberg EO. (2006). *Redefining Health Care: Creating Value-Based Competition on Results.* Harvard Business School Press, Boston.

Reinhardt UE. (2004). "The Swiss health system. Regulated competition without managed care." *J Am Med Assoc* **292**(10): 1227–1231.

Schut FT, Gress S, Wasem J. (2003). "Consumer price sensitivity and social health insurer choice in Germany and The Netherlands." *Int J Health Care Fin Econ* **3**(2): 117–138.

SFSO. (2005). *Coût et Financement du Système de Santé en 2003* ["The Swiss health expenditure and financing in 2003"]. Office Fédéral de la Statistique, Neuchâtel.

SFSO. (2006). *Coût et Financement du Système de Santé en 2004* ["The Swiss health expenditure and financing in 2004"]. Office Fédéral de la Statistique, Neuchâtel.

Strombom BA, Buchmueller TC, Feldstein PJ. (2002). "Switching costs, price sensitivity and health plan choice." *J Health Econ* **21**(1): 89–116.

Swiss Federal Council. (2004). "Message du Conseil Fédéral du 26 Mai 2004 Relatif à la Révision Partielle de la Loi Fédérale Sur l'Assurance-Maladie (Stratégie et Thèmes Urgents)" ["Message of the Federal Council Regarding the Partial Revision of the Federal Law on Health Insurance of 26 March 2004"]. Accessed 23 February 2009. www.admin.ch/ch/f/ff/2004/4019.pdf.

Swiss Federal Council. (2005). "Message du Conseil Fédéral du 22 Juin 2005 Concernant l'Initiative Populaire. Pour Une Baisse des Primes d'Assurance-Maladie Dans l'Assurance de Base" ["Message of the Federal Council Regarding the Popular Initiative to Reduce the Premiums of the Basic Health Insurance of 22 June 2005"]. Accessed date 23 February 2009. www.admin. ch/ch/f/ff/2005/4095.pdf.

Swiss Federal Council. (2005). "Message du Conseil Fédéral du 9 Décembre 2005 Concernant l'Initiative Populaire. Pour Une Caisse Maladie Unique et Sociale" ["Message of the Federal Council Regarding the Popular Initiative for a National Health Insurance Fund"]. Accessed 23 February 2009. www.admin. ch/ch/f/ff/2006/725.pdf.

Teisberg EO. (2008). *Nutzenorientierter Wettbewerb im Schweizerischen Gesundheitswesen: Möglichkeiten und Chancen* ["A Value-based competition perspective for the Swiss health care system"]. Publikation von Economiesuisse, Zürich.

Tiebout CM. (1956). "A pure theory of local expenditures." *J Polit Econ* **64**(5): 416–424.

Van Doorslaer E, Masseria C, Koolman X. (2006). "Inequalities in access to medical care by income in developed countries." *Can Med Assoc J* **174**(2): 177–183.

Van Doorslaer E, Koolman X, Puffer F. (2002). "Equity in the use of physicians in the OECD countries: Has equal treatment for equal need been achieved?" In: *Measuring Up: Health Systems Performance in OECD Countries*, ed. OECD. OECD, Paris.

Wagstaff A *et al.* (1999). "Equity in the finance of health care: Some further international comparisons." *J Health Econ* **18**(3): 263–290.

WHO. (2000). *The World Health Report 2000. Health Systems: Improving Performance*. World Health Organization, Geneva.

Zweifel P. (2004). "Competition in health care — the Swiss experience." *Économie Publique* **14**(1): 3–12.

Zweifel P, Telser H, Vaterlaus S. (2006). "Consumer resistance against regulation: The case of health care." *J Regul Econ* **29**(3): 319–332.

Chapter 6

Taiwan's National Health Insurance System: High Value for the Dollar

*Tsung-Mei Cheng**

Introduction

Taiwan is a relatively high-income democracy of 23 million people, with a per capita GNP of US$17,299 in 2007 (calculated at the market exchange rate of ~NT$1 equals US$0.03), or US$30,100 if measured in purchasing power parity (PPP) (Department of Health [DoH], 2009; International Monetary Fund, 2007). Taiwan established a universal national health insurance scheme — National Health Insurance (NHI) — on 1 March 1995. Today, this government-operated single-payer system provides health insurance to 99% of Taiwan's population.

The NHI's benefit package is very comprehensive. It includes inpatient and outpatient care, dental care, prescription drugs, and even traditional Chinese medicine (TCM). In 2007, these broad benefits were available to Taiwan's population at a total national expenditure from all sources of 6.13% of the gross domestic product (GDP) (DoH, 2008).

The NHI does not cover long-term care. Out-of-pocket spending by households accounted for 37% of total health care spending in Taiwan in 2007 (DoH, 2008), which is high by Organization for Economic Cooperation and Development (OECD) standards. Cost sharing by patients includes copayments and coinsurance for covered services, which have been increasing in recent years. Out-of-pocket spending also

* International Forum, Princeton University, USA. Email: maycrein@princeton.edu.

includes services not covered by the NHI, such as orthodontics, prosthodontics, extra charges for private and semiprivate rooms, special nurses, and nursing home care. Consequently, the NHI itself now accounts for only 53% of total national health spending (Cheng, 2003; DoH, 2008). Overall, however, Taiwan's citizens enjoy access to a broad set of health care benefits at costs that are moderate by international standards.

Moreover, population-wide satisfaction rates with the NHI are very high by international standards. As of July 2008, over 77% of surveyed individuals declared themselves satisfied with Taiwan's NHI (BNHI, 2007). At the same time, by international standards, Taiwan's health statistics are commendable, too. As of 2007, the infant mortality rate was 4.98 per 1000 live births compared to more than 7 per 1000 live births in the United States, and life expectancy at birth is 82 years for women and 75 years for men (DoH, 2009).

This chapter describes Taiwan's experience with national health insurance from its beginning to today. We will see that a determined and strong government can, indeed, implement major change in social policy. The chapter will also show that such a program begets a variety of politically powerful stakeholders on both the supply and demand side of the system. While the government allowed providers very limited time and opportunities to give their input during the planning and implementation stages of the NHI in the years from the mid-1980s to 1995, just a few years after the NHI's implementation the same providers had become a formidable voice in Taiwan's health policy as the democratization process matured in Taiwan. The government found itself faced with strong and determined opposition from organized groups against numerous policy initiatives. For example, it faced strong opposition from Taiwan's hospitals when it sought to amend provider payment schemes from the current fee-for-service payment to payment by diagnostic-related groups (DRGs). Similarly, in 2002, the government faced such strong opposition from the public and their political representatives when it sought to increase copayments and coinsurance that it had to rescind the decision.

A Brief History of Health Insurance in Taiwan

Before the implementation of the NHI in 1995, Taiwan had 13 different health insurance schemes, each covering a subset of the population. For example, Labor Insurance covered private sector workers, Government Employees Insurance covered public sector workers including teachers, Farmers Insurance covered farmers, and so on. Together, those insurance schemes covered almost 59% of the population (Cheng, 2003). However, the remaining 41% of the population, including vulnerable groups like children under 14, women, the elderly, and the disabled — those who had the greatest need for health insurance — were not covered by any health insurance scheme. Medical bills frequently impoverished patients and their families (as still happens in the U.S. today), and even those who had insurance worried about medical expenses for the members of their family without health insurance.

By the 1980s, things began to change, as Taiwan's policy-makers responded to several factors that created a "window of opportunity" (Kingdon, 1984) for fundamental reform. First, buoyed by robust economic growth, which averaged more than 8% a year from the early 1950s to the 1980s, the public started to expect a higher quality of life, including improved health care and improved financial protection from the cost of illness. At the same time, the lifting in 1987 of the martial law that had been imposed on Taiwan since 1949 by the long-ruling Kuomintang (KMT) government ushered in a period of political liberalization that saw the emergence of an organized and increasingly vocal and influential political opposition: the Democratic Progressive Party (DPP). The KMT had been in power since the Chinese government retreated to Taiwan from the mainland in 1949, after losing the civil war to the Communists.

As the DPP began to compete openly for political power with the KMT, the latter, at least in part to safeguard its power, set about establishing a universal national health insurance scheme that would cover the entire population, as most of the wealthy Western democracies and Japan had done for their people (with the exception of the U.S.). Taiwan's then KMT president, Lee Teng-hui, himself orchestrated the massive undertaking. From a historical perspective, this experience was similar to the passage of social health insurance in Germany in the late 19th century: worried about the rise of the labor movement, the conservative Chancellor Bismarck introduced social insurance schemes for industrial workers as a pre-emptive strike. In Germany, it was a pre-emptive strike against the growing political power of socialism. In Taiwan, it was a pre-emptive strike against the growing political power of the opposition DPP. In both cases, the moves to reform can be viewed as a mixture of paternalistic concern for the welfare of the people, amplified by self-serving political interests.

Planning for the NHI scheme took seven-and-a-half years, from the mid-1980s through the early 1990s. The government engaged foreign experts to advise on the reform process and options, and also sent its officials and researchers abroad to study foreign schemes and experiences (Cheng, 2003). The planning stage was followed by 18 months of intense lobbying by government officials to pass the NHI into law. Once again, President Lee Teng-hui personally took charge of that effort, aided by his premier, Lien Chan and deputy premier, Hsu Li-de. Lobbying often lasted into the wee hours of the night. Eventually, on 19 July 1994, Parliament passed the NHI Law (Cheng, 2003).

The NHI Law originally called for the implementation of the NHI by 2000, allowing for a five-year phase-in. Impatient with that long a wait, however, President Lee decreed that the NHI was to be implemented fully in 1995, an amazing five years ahead of schedule. Great uncertainty and opposition, including from physicians, surrounded the president's decision. Many felt that the plan was not yet ready for implementation and feared that, if prematurely implemented, the plan would fail before it had a chance to work.

The president and his government did not waver. Under the tight time schedule between Parliament's passage of the NHI Law in July 1994 and the implementation date of 1 March 1995, Taiwan's providers were given a three-day consultation period to give feedback, from 26 to 28 February 1995. Implementation took place on 1 March 1995, as scheduled. Chaos followed, and providers were in shock. Nevertheless, by the end of 1995, the NHI covered 90% of the population (Yeh, 2002), and public satisfaction with the NHI reached 70% (Yeh, 2007). By 2003, the NHI covered 99% of the population (Chang, 2005).

History may well have shown that pushing up the implementation of the NHI a full five years was a smart move. In 1997, the Asian financial crisis struck. Although Taiwan was not directly hit by that crisis as some of the other Asian economies, economic growth nevertheless slowed from 1998 through the 2000s; in 2001, Taiwan suffered a negative growth rate of −2.22% as a result of the bursting of the dot-com bubble in 2000 (DoH, 2005). Had Taiwan waited until 2000 to implement the NHI, as specified by the NHI Law, the NHI might never have seen the light of day because of concerns over affordability and financial sustainability (Cheng, 2003).

Administration of the NHI

Taiwan's NHI is a single-payer social health insurance scheme administered by the Bureau of National Health Insurance (BNHI) under the Department of Health (DoH). Unlike the single-payer British National Health Service (NHS), or the single-payer schemes of some other European countries where the government acts as both the insurer and the predominant provider of services, Taiwan's single-payer NHI acts as the sole insurer, and leaves the provision of services to a largely private delivery system. The NHI thus combines a public insurance system that offers universal and equitable access to health care with a predominantly private delivery system that provides the competition which a public delivery system often lacks. Some policy analysts have attributed the success of the NHI to this feature of the program.

Taiwan's health policy pursues three major social goals: first, preserving social solidarity and equity in access to needed health care; second, promoting high-quality health care; and third, promoting cost-effectiveness — the greatest benefit for a given outlay of resources, or, alternatively, minimizing the cost of a given outcome (Cheng, 2008).

Taiwan's BNHI is indeed a lean and efficient organization — perhaps too lean. Its administrative budget was a mere 1.5% in 2007. With a staff of 3072, including 517 temporary workers, it administers the NHI through six regional offices for Taiwan's 23 million people (BNHI, 2008). The BNHI performs many functions: collecting premiums, processing claims, paying providers, conducting medical reviews, monitoring utilization, doing research and development that aims to promote the quality and efficiency of the system (such as payment system reforms and health information technology), and managing public relations. The public relations function covers the NHI's interface with providers of care, patient advocacy groups, individual patients, lobbying groups, the media, and, last but not least, the U.S. Trade Representative, which fronts U.S. business interest under the mantle of the World Trade Organization (WTO). As a member of the WTO, Taiwan's government is obligated to address trade-related issues, such as prices of pharmaceuticals and medical devices, which, in turn, impact Taiwan's national health policy. These responsibilities fall to the BNHI, as the operational arm of the government's national health policy.

Financing of the NHI

Taiwan's NHI is a premium-based system that derives its funding from three sources: households (38%), employers (37%), and government (25%). Because these premiums are mandated by the government, they technically are a form of (earmarked) taxes. Households and breadwinners' employers pay premiums to the NHI, and the government subsidizes the contributions of particular population subgroups. Figure 1 illustrates how the three parties share the costs of the NHI.

In recent years, the share of premiums paid by Taiwan's government in the form of subsidies has been declining gradually, from 30% in 2001 (DoH, 2008) to 28% in 2005 (DoH, 2008), and to 25% in 2007 (DoH, 2008). This is (in part) due to growing government deficits in the past several years. As a result, household out-of-pocket spending in Taiwan has been increasing, from 32% in 2002 (Cheng, 2003) to the current 37% of total health spending, considerably higher than for many countries in the OECD. The average household out-of-pocket spending for developed countries is usually below 20% (OECD, 2006). Among the 27 countries a

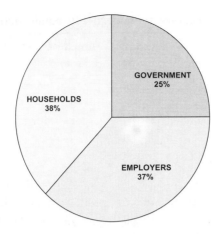

Source: Based on data from the Department of Health's *2006 Health Statistical Trends.*

Fig. 1. Sources of premium revenue 2007 of Taiwan's NHI: Who writes the checks to the Bureau of National Health Insurance?

U.S. congressional study examined, only South Korea, Greece, and Mexico have higher out-of-pocket spending than Taiwan (Peterson, 2007). Some policy analysts in Taiwan fear a gradual erosion of equity and the corresponding decrease in access to care if the trend of growing out-of-pocket spending is not reversed.

For the purpose of assessing and collecting premiums, the BNHI divides Taiwan's 23-million population — the insured — into six population categories, such as the employed, the self-employed, union workers, farmers, fishermen, the indigent, and veterans, and so on. What premium an insured pays depends on his or her population category status. Varying amounts of government subsidies, from 0 to 100%, apply to the six population categories. Table 1 shows the relative shares of premiums paid by each of the three sources of financing for the six population categories under the NHI. The BNHI collects premiums from the insured at a rate of 4.55% of the wages or salary on a monthly basis (see Table 1). For families with an employed breadwinner, employers share in these premiums. At present, up to a maximum of NT$131,700 (US$4046) of the monthly salary and wages are subject to assessment for premium levying, at the

Table 1. Sources of Taiwan's NHI Premium Contribution

"Population Category"	Insured* (%)	Employer (%)	Government (%)	Population (%)
1st	Private-sector employees	30	60	10	53.01
	Government employees	30	70	—	
	Self-employed, employers	100	—	—	
2nd	Union workers	60	—	40	16.67
3rd	Farmers, fishermen	30	—	70	13.73
4th	Military personnel	—	—	100	NA
5th	Low-income households	—	—	100	0.97
6th	Veterans or	—	—	100	15.61
	Survivors of veterans	30	—	70	
	"Community population"	60	—	40	

* Dependents and the insured in category 6 must be unemployed.

Source: Bureau of National Health Insurance. 2007. *National Health Insurance in Taiwan — Profile 2007*. Taipei: Bureau of National Health Insurance.

rate of 4.55%. Any additional earnings from the salary and wages are exempted from premium levying. For military and public sector employees, including teachers, 87% of their total compensation is assessed for premium contributions, at the 4.55% rate (BNHI, 2008). For the aborigines in Taiwan (constituting 1.45% of Taiwan's population), the government subsidizes the premiums for those under 20 years and over 55 years of age and who are unemployed.

Premiums are levied on a per capita basis. This means, for example, that for a family with an employed breadwinner and two dependents, a total contribution of three (persons) times 4.55% of the breadwinner's wage or salary is levied, while for a household of four, four (persons) times 4.55% of the breadwinner's salary or wage is levied — shared, as noted above, by employer, employee, and by government, where applicable (see Table 1). The maximum number of dependents per household is capped at three; any members of the household above four are automatically insured free of charge. Since 2008, premiums and bona-fide out-of-pocket medical expenses have been deductible from income taxes.

The NHI's cumbersome premium structure at times invites criticism for its complexity and built-in biases because of the different subsidy schemes applied to the different categories of the insured, as shown in Table 1 (DoH, 2007). For example, the self-employed receive no government subsidy, even though many among its ranks earn modest incomes. On the other hand, many individuals may earn salaries or wages significantly above the ceiling set for the assessable salary or wages of NT$131,700, but pay no premium on their wage or salary earnings above that ceiling.

Taiwan's NHI combines several features of the traditional European social health insurance schemes (see the introduction to this book), whose most important feature is universal access. In the U.S., individuals who do not have employer-provided health insurance coverage at work or access to public health insurance programs such as Medicare or Medicaid may procure health insurance in the commercial nongroup insurance market, but their acceptance by private health insurance carriers is by no means guaranteed. Pre-existing conditions preclude many Americans from obtaining private health insurance altogether, as private health insurers, understandably, are reluctant to cover individuals who represent bad risks to the company's bottom line. And private insurance carriers may ask for exceedingly high premiums for policies with limited coverage to high-risk individuals. Sometimes privately insured individuals are dropped from private coverage altogether following a recent episode of illness. By contrast, in Taiwan, a person's health status or pre-existing condition has no bearing whatsoever on the amount of contribution he or she pays, and health insurance coverage is guaranteed from cradle to grave. In addition, unlike in the UK, where the NHS has implicit upper limits on the cost per quality adjusted life year (QALY) it is willing to pay to extend life (currently around £30,000), Taiwan's NHI does not (yet) have a ceiling on what insurance will pay for saving or extending life (LeGrand, 2003; Devlin *et al.*, 2003). Finally, Taiwan's NHI does not allow balance billing by providers, assuring full equity in the services received by all insured, regardless of their economic station in life. Providers are paid fees for their services set by the BNHI, and are not allowed to charge more than what the NHI fee schedule pays for covered services.

Very recently, however, the BNHI has begun to make a few exceptions to the general rule of no balance billing. Patients are now allowed to buy more expensive versions of certain devices and pay the difference in cost between the standard device that is covered by the BNHI (such as bare metal stents, standard intraocular lens implants following cataract surgery, and metal artificial knees) and the more expensive versions of the same type of device (such as drug-eluting stents, pricier kinds of intraocular lens implants, and ceramic artificial knees). Under this new policy, the BNHI helps patients become educated consumers by publishing on the Internet and in print media the prices of different devices, by type and by hospital. For example, the BNHI publishes the prices different hospitals charge for all the different types of intraocular lens implants that are available in Taiwan but are not covered by the NHI. Armed with this information, patients are thus enabled, and indeed encouraged, by the BNHI to compare prices before the procedure. Should they choose to have the non-NHI-covered lens implant, they pay only the difference between the special lens of their choice and the NHI-covered lens. This is, indeed, a real-life example of "consumer-driven health care" based on usable information. Patients are enabled to "shop around" for what they deem to be the best care for them.

Cost Sharing by Patients

Patients in Taiwan pay copayments and coinsurance for inpatient and outpatient care, dental care, traditional Chinese medicine, and drugs. So as not to impair patients' access to necessary care, exemptions are made for special circumstances. In such cases, patients receive first-dollar coverage without having to pay copayment and coinsurance (BNHI, 2008). Exemptions are stipulated in Article 36 of the NHI Law, and include 30 major diseases and conditions (cancer, hemophilia, chronic mental illness, polio, etc.), childbirth, preventative care, care in hospitals and clinics in remote, mountainous areas and offshore islands, veterans, low-income households, patients who suffer from occupational diseases, tuberculosis patients, and children under the age of three whose care is paid for by other government agencies. Persons with physical and mental disabilities pay a uniform copayment of NT$50 (US$1.50) across the board. Furthermore, outpatient services that are within the DRG payment scheme and patients who are on prescription medications for chronic conditions or illnesses are exempted from copayments and coinsurance (BNHI, 2008). Coinsurance rates for hospital stays for acute and chronic illnesses average between 5% and 10% for average length stays, with higher coinsurance rates for longer stays to discourage overuse (BNHI, 2008). There are ceilings for total annual outlays by the insured of copayments and coinsurance, however, to limit the impact on a household's finances. The Department of Health makes annual public announcements about the ceilings (BNHI, 2008).

Finally, since the inception of the NHI, providers have been permitted by the BNHI to charge registration fees for each patient contact with either an outpatient (clinics and hospital outpatient departments) or inpatient facility. These registration fees are akin to cover charges in European restaurants. One pays them just to be registered for a visit with a medical provider, or for hospital admission. Table 2 provides an illustration of the different registration fees currently charged by different types of providers. Note that the registration fees charged by primary care clinics may be higher than those charged by medical centers, and there are large variations in the registration fees charged by public hospitals under the jurisdiction of the DoH. There have been several increases in the

Table 2. Registration Fees in Taiwan's NHI, 2008 (in NT$)

Medical centers	50–250
Medical centers, ER	80–700
DoH public hospitals	10–20
DoH public hospitals, ER	120–500
Regional hospitals	180–380
Regional hospitals, ER	300–900
Primary care clinics	100–400

Source: Lin, J. Y. 2008. "Registration Fees Annual Profit 500 Yi — Uncontrollable." *United Daily Evening News*, 24 January.

registration fees over time. In 2008, higher registration fees were charged at a time when oil and consumer prices rose sharply, resulting in hardship for many in Taiwan. The DoH has been called upon to conduct a thorough investigation to determine the standards used by providers in setting registration fees, and to establish standardization of registration fees.

Health Care Delivery in Taiwan

Health care services in Taiwan are delivered through a predominantly private delivery system, like under Canada's provincial single-payer Medicare plans, or the Dutch health system (see chapter on The Netherlands). Seventy percent of Taiwan's hospital beds are private, and 53% of all doctors work in private clinics. The rest of Taiwan's doctors work in hospitals, many of which are private.

Bed occupancy in Taiwan averages 66.3%, suggesting overcapacity; but the figure is misleading, because there is a wide discrepancy between the very high bed occupancy rates in large hospitals (especially medical centers where beds are much in demand and waiting lists are long) and the much lower rates in small and medium-size hospitals. Over time, the trend for the hospital sector has been towards ever greater concentration of resources and delivery of services in large hospitals, especially in medical centers where high-tech medicine is available. As of 2005, Taiwan's 15 largest hospitals accounted for 32% of the total hospital work force and 44% of all hospital-based physicians (DoH, 2006). In addition, the 15 largest hospitals performed 31% of all surgical procedures (both ambulatory and inpatient surgery) in Taiwan (DoH, 2006).

Indeed, while the total number of beds has increased rapidly since the implementation of the NHI, many small and medium-size hospitals in Taiwan have closed their doors or reduced their number of beds. Small and medium-size hospitals simply are not in a position to compete with the large hospitals for resources, and thus cannot adequately compete for patients. If one were to look at the distribution of health care resources by provider type, one would observe what people in Taiwan call

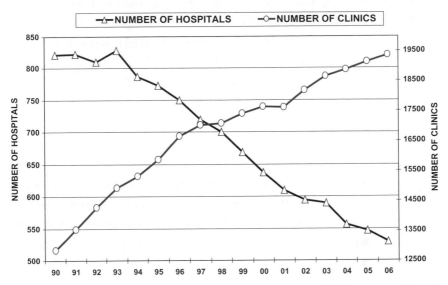

Source: Department of Health. 2008. *2007 Health Statistical Trends*. Taipei: Department of Health, the Executive Yuan.

Fig. 2. Changes in the number of hospitals and clinics in Taiwan 1990–2006.

the "M-shape" distribution curve, with the two extremes showing the decrease in the total number of hospitals and the increase in the total number of primary care clinics, respectively (DoH, 2008). Figure 2 provides a graphic illustration of this trend. In the decade between 1997 and 2007, the number of hospitals in Taiwan decreased by 29%, while the number of clinics increased by 16% (DoH, 2008).

Choice of Providers

Patients in Taiwan enjoy complete free choice of providers. There are no waiting lists, in contrast to other single-payer systems, such as the UK's NHS or Canada's Medicare. Nor is there a gatekeeper system like that in the NHS (or, for that matter, like the Dutch multipayer system) under which general practitioners act as gatekeepers and refer and triage patients elsewhere for services.

In recent years, however, Taiwan's government has been trying to establish a referral system in their continuing attempt to achieve a more rational use of resources. Thus, in July 2005, the BNHI introduced a voluntary referral scheme whereby patients referred to a higher-level-of-care institution make a lower copayment than those who go directly to a higher-level-of-care provider without referral. For example, if a patient goes directly to a medical center without being referred by either a primary care physician or a local or regional hospital, that patient is charged a copayment of NT$360 (US$11) for the visit, whereas with a referral the patient is charged the considerably lower copayment of NT$210 (US$6). In the end, though, freedom of choice of providers appears to be so entrenched in Taiwan's national psyche that moving away from that tradition would be a monumental task, or even a "mission impossible." Complete free choice of providers is viewed as a right by patients in Taiwan.

The Taiwanese frequently use their health care system. In 2007, a person in Taiwan made, on average, 12 visits (office visits at clinics and visits to hospital outpatient departments for ambulatory care) per year (BNHI, 2008). In 2001, the BNHI implemented a plan to deal with abnormally high users of the NHI in order to create greater efficiency in resource utilization and to encourage patients to take greater responsibility for appropriate care. "High users" are those patients identified by the BNHI as having made more than either 150 outpatient visits in the previous year (before March 2007, the maximum was 200 visits in the previous year), 50 outpatient visits in the first quarter of any year, or 20 outpatient visits per month (BNHI, 2008). The NHI's powerful IT system identifies the high users easily.

High users are treated gently by the BNHI. The BNHI uses one or a combination of the following methods to guide high users toward more appropriate usage: a personal visit or telephone call by a BNHI case worker to inquire whether the patient has difficulty getting care or medication; a friendly letter to the patient with information on the various services the BNHI provides that may be helpful to the patient's particular needs, along with contact information of personnel at appropriate provider organizations where the patient may seek care; a review of the patient's medical records by specialists to determine both the appropriateness of care the patient has been given and whether the high number of visits can be justified — such information is then forwarded to the patient's provider(s) to help reduce the frequency of visits and raise the quality of care the patient receives from those providers; enlistment of the help of multiple other government agencies, such as the local public health office, the Veterans Administration, or trained volunteers; and finally, as a last resort, specifying which providers the patient may visit henceforth — thus taking away the patient's right of free choice of providers (BNHI, 2008).

This set of measures has yielded impressive results. As of June 2007, the number of visits per capita among "high users" was reduced by an average of 30–60%, depending on the length of time the patient had been under the BNHI's gentle "guidance." Often, the problems plaguing high users are not medical in nature and can be remedied by counseling or help that can easily be obtained from other, non-NHI sources.

Contracting with and Paying the Providers of Care

Providers in Taiwan deliver services through contractual agreement with the BNHI. Currently, 92% of all Taiwan's providers contract with the BNHI (BNHI, 2008). The BNHI payments constitute the largest part of providers' income. Other sources of income include patient registration fees, copayments and coinsurance, and profits from sale of products and services not covered by the NHI, like cosmetic surgery or orthodontics.

Fee-for-service (FFS) payment, which varies by the level of provider within each category of provider, has remained the predominant payment method of the NHI since its inception. These fees are set by the government — as they are by the U.S. single-payer federal Medicare program for the elderly — and not formally negotiated between the government and associations of providers, as is the case in many European countries.

To set its fees, the NHI groups providers into four levels of service provision. At the top, assigned and receiving the highest fees, are medical centers. Next are regional hospitals, then local hospitals, and finally, at the lowest level, outpatient clinics. All providers at the same provider level receive the same payment for the same service. This approach to payment was adopted by the NHI because, according to Lee Cheng-hua, MD, a Vice President of the BNHI, "different levels of provider organizations go by different operating standards, for example, square meters allowed per bed, ratios of physicians to beds, the availability of specialties and subspecialties, all of which give rise to different cost structures for the different levels of provider organizations" (Lee, 2008).[1] Horizontal equity in payment is preserved for all providers at the same level of provider organization.

Patients also enjoy equal treatment at the hands of their providers under this payment system when they seek care within the same level of provider organization, since all providers at that particular level of provider organization receive the same fees for their service, regardless of the patient's socioeconomic status. By contrast, in the U.S., a provider receives a much lower fee for a particular service when the patient is covered by the public Medicaid program for the poor than if that provider were to perform the same service for a patient that was commercially insured. Low fees paid by Medicaid have led many physicians to refuse to treat Medicaid patients altogether. In effect, the U.S. payment system signals to health care providers that the value of their services varies by the social class of the patient. This would be viewed as unacceptable in Taiwan, as in many other countries. Remarkably, it has long been the norm in the U.S.

Traditionally, hospitals in Taiwan have been paid on a FFS basis, which continued even under the sectoral global budget for hospitals that began in 2002. Unfortunately, inherent in any FFS payment system is the incentive for providers to induce demand. Taiwan's NHI is no exception. Like payers in many other countries, the BNHI has developed other payment methods in an attempt to achieve higher efficiency and quality for the care it procures from providers. For example, in recent years, the BNHI has sought to shift the payment scheme for hospitals to a case-based (DRG) method. So far, it has implemented 53 DRGs for inpatient

---

[1] Verbal communication from Vice President Lee Cheng-hua of the BNHI during a meeting with the author. Taipei, Taiwan. March 2008.

services (BNHI, 2006). Unfortunately, provider resistance has repeatedly delayed full implementation of a DRG system for Taiwan's hospital sector (see also the chapters on Israel and The Netherlands). In addition, patient advocacy groups have voiced concerns about providers possibly withholding services, including dumping patients, if they were paid by DRGs, despite the fact that the DRG or case payment approach has not led to serious problems of this nature in other countries where they are used.

The BNHI has also experimented with case payments based on the quality and outcomes of care given patients. The scheme is akin to the pay-for-performance (P4P) scheme used in numerous countries. In stages, beginning in October 2001, it chose five diseases and chronic conditions — cervical cancer (replaced by hypertension in 2006), breast cancer, tuberculosis, diabetes, and asthma — for the experimental P4P scheme. Provider participation in the programs is voluntary. In 2006, patient enrollment in the various P4P schemes ranged between 7.79% for hypertension and 78.99% for tuberculosis (BNHI, 2008). To date, available data on the results of the experiments with P4P in terms of input, process, and outcome appear encouraging. For example, the one-year survival rate for breast cancer patients is higher for patients enrolled in the breast cancer P4P program than for those who are not. Satisfaction among the enrolled breast cancer patients is more than 90%. For enrolled diabetes patients, there has been a marked improvement in clinical indicators such as fasting glucose levels (BNHI, 2008).

Cost Containment Through Global Budgets

For all but the first three years (1995–1998) of the NHI's 13-year history, premium revenue has fallen short of expenditure. Figure 3 illustrates the financial situation of the NHI from 1995 through 2007, including when it experienced its first financial crisis in 2002 (DoH, 2008). A one-time premium rate increase, from 4.25% to 4.55% (a 7% increase), resolved the financial shortfall through December 2004. At the same time, the government implemented a global budget for the hospital sector whereby all of Taiwan's hospitals were brought under one common budget, which is

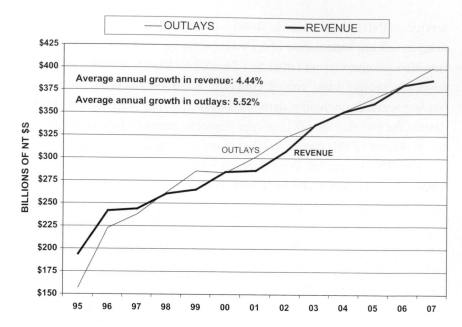

Source: Department of Health. 2008. *2007 Health Statistical Trends.* Taipei: Department of Health, Executive Yuan.

Fig. 3. Revenues and outlays of Taiwan's NHI, 1995–2007.

reviewed and revised annually by the government with inputs from the different stakeholders.

The original design of the NHI had actually called for global budgeting, to be implemented five years after the NHI's implementation as a way to contain costs (Cheng, 2003). Accordingly, the BNHI had implemented global budgets, by sector, beginning with dental care in 1999, traditional Chinese medicine in 2000, and primary care in 2001. Finally, the imposition of the hospital global budget in 2002 by the government brought the vast hospital sector under one overall hospital global budget. In 2003, the BNHI implemented a fifth sectoral global budget, for hemodialysis, perhaps in response to the high prevalence of diabetes among Taiwan's population.

Although sectoral global budgets are not the ideal long-term solution to the health system's financial problems, so far they remain the working solution for cost containment in Taiwan's NHI. By now, providers have learned to live with these global budgets; doctors and administrators in the hospital global sector have accepted lower pay, longer work hours, and more frugal working conditions, like higher temperatures in operating rooms (Cheng, 2008).[2] Interestingly, among dentists and doctors of traditional Chinese medicine, satisfaction is high with their respective global budgets.

The NHI's Health Information System

Taiwan's NHI could not have performed all of the functions demanded of it without the support of the powerful information technology (IT) system it has built over time. Taiwan's health IT system is considered superior even to that of Denmark, currently ranked number one among the most advanced OECD countries (Pedersen, 2007).[3]

Patients in Taiwan access health care with the NHI integrated circuitry (IC) card, which is issued to every insured resident. The credit-card-size card stores basic personal information, such as name, date of birth, gender, and personal national ID number, and also records serious illness and injury (with effective starting and ending dates), prescriptions, allergies, and major examinations, such as CT, MRI, and PET imaging. As discussed earlier, patients in Taiwan are exempted from paying copayments and coinsurance if they have any of the 30 exempted diseases and conditions — recording a patient's circumstances on their NHI IC card provides proof of their condition. The card also records the last six visits the patient made and the diagnoses (in designated codes) established during those visits, and enables easy preauthorization of certain expensive high-tech procedures — such as CT, MRI, and PET scans — for purposes of cost containment.

[2] Verbal communication from meetings with physicians and hospital administrators of the National Taiwan University Hospital, Jen-Ai Municipal Hospital, and Chang-Gung Memorial Hospital, and Taipei, Taiwan. April 2007.
[3] Panel remarks by Kjeld Pedersen at a session on health information technology in Taiwan's National Health Insurance. 5th International Health Economics Association World Congress. Copenhagen, Denmark. 10 July 2007.

In addition, the card records the premium payment history, which serves as a convenient reminder to the cardholder of his or her premium payment status, and when premiums are next due. Premium payment may be made through automatic bank transfers or by paying in person at 24-hour electronic kiosks, convenience stores like 7–Eleven, and the post office. A total of 98% of Taiwanese pay premiums on time (BNHI, 2007).

At the beginning of any visit, the patient swipes his or her IC card through the provider's patient card reader, which immediately registers the patient's contact with the health care system in the BNHI's vast database. Thus, the BNHI is automatically and immediately made aware of the visit. Next, the provider swipes his or her own provider ID card through the provider card reader, a step that immediately links the provider with the particular patient in the BNHI's information system. Finally, the provider begins to deliver care to the patient, and bills the BNHI electronically for the services delivered.

Thus, the BNHI can know virtually in real time what service is being delivered to which patient by which provider at what care institution at what time on what day. For example, it can know that patient X had his third molar extracted at dentist Y's office at 10 a.m. on Monday, 18 June 2008. Such precise information gathering in real time is a powerful tool in utilization monitoring and fraud detection (Lee, 2008)[4]; indeed, the BNHI uses the IT system to detect potential overuse and abuse of the NHI by both providers (induced demand) and patients (patient demand). Furthermore, each provider is required to deliver a daily service log, by patient and by service, to the BNHI every 24 hours. This enables the BNHI to keep track of the total volume of services provided by each individual provider and each care institution. It also allows the BNHI to know the total volume of services delivered at any one point in time by all the providers.

---

[4] Verbal communication from Vice President Lee Cheng-hua of the BNHI during a meeting with the author. Taipei, Taiwan. May 2008.

Under the global budgets, all services are assigned relative-value units (RVUs) for the purpose of fee-for-service payment. For example, an ambulatory visit at a hospital outpatient department may receive a hypothetical 250 RVUs. Under the constraint of a global budget, the dollar value per RVU naturally fluctuates inversely with the total volume of services delivered within a certain period of time — say, a month. The higher the volume of services delivered, the lower the dollar value per RVU paid by the BNHI. Because information on the volume of services delivered by providers is known virtually in real time, the BNHI can continuously update the NT$ of the "relative point unit" (*dian zhi*) of all the services delivered on a fee-for-service basis under the sectoral global budgets.

At the end of each predetermined interval within the calendar year — say, a month or quarter — the RVUs accumulated by all the hospitals are added up, and then the total is divided by the total hospital global budget for that period to arrive at the dollar value per RVU for all the services delivered during that period. Providers are paid according to the total volume of services they provided during that period multiplied by the price per RVU for that period. Thus the global budgets can be met automatically through an automatic reduction in the NT$ value of fees, should the actual volume exceed the budgeted volume.

With such a powerful information system, patient privacy naturally is a major concern of the BNHI (Lee, 2008).[5] Extensive scrambling of recorded patient information by the BNHI helps insure data security. Thus far, the public has not taken issue with the way the NHI IC card is used; satisfaction with the card is extremely high. Public health authorities, such as Taiwan's Center for Disease Control and Prevention, also use the database to look for unusual patterns of NHI service utilization that may point to local epidemics or even pandemics, such as SARS and the avian flu. Finally, the NHI database could provide the roots for a system of more comprehensive electronic personal records in the future.

---

[5] Verbal communication from Vice President Lee Cheng-hua of the BNHI during a meeting with the author. Taipei, Taiwan. March 2008.

The Role of the State and Organized Stakeholders in Taiwan's Health Policy

To appreciate the role of the state in Taiwan's health reform, one must bear in mind the different phases Taiwan's young democracy has traveled in recent history. The official "birth" of Taiwan's democracy took place in 1987, when the long-ruling Kuomintang (KMT) government abolished the martial law that had been in place since 1949, the year the KMT government retreated from the Chinese mainland across the Taiwan Strait to the island of Taiwan following its defeat by the Chinese communists in the civil war. For 50 years, between 1949 and 2000, Taiwan was ruled by three strong KMT leaders in succession: Chiang Kai-shek (president 1950–1975); Chiang Kai-shek's son, Chiang Ching-kuo (premier 1972–1978, president 1978–1988); and Lee Teng-hui (vice president 1984–1988, president 1988–2000). Under Chiang Kai-shek's authoritarian government, citizens had limited political and civil freedoms, such as free speech. Dissidents were considered supporters of either the Chinese communists or the Taiwan Independence movement, and were often imprisoned. Under Chiang Ching-kuo, the public enjoyed much greater civil liberties, including greater rights of political dissent; further, native Taiwanese representation increased in the government at every level, including Parliament. In fact, Chiang Ching-kuo's handpicked successor and Taiwan's eventual president, Lee Teng-hui is a native Taiwanese. A major achievement of President Lee Teng-hui's administration was the implementation of the NHI in 1995.

Against this political backdrop, it is easy to understand how Taiwan was able to achieve universal national health insurance in a relatively short period of time. During the formative years of the young democracy, powerful organized interest groups such as those in older democracies like the U.S., Japan, or Germany did not yet exist, and the government had a much freer hand to do as it saw fit. Witness the treatment of physicians by Taiwan's government in the days before the implementation of the NHI — they were not extensively consulted during the planning and implementation of the new NHI program. Despite the fact that, at that time, physicians enjoyed an exalted status in Taiwan's society, they did not have much de facto power in the political affairs of the government. This stands in sharp contrast to their colleagues in the U.S., and in many other countries.

As democracy matured in Taiwan, health policy became much more of a political football than it had been in the past. Organized interest groups in health care, such as physician specialty associations, hospital associations, associations of drug and device manufacturers, patient advocacy groups, and NGOs like the Federation of NHI Public Oversight and the Association of Medical Reform (*Yi Gai Hui*) were formed and began to exert considerable pressure and influence on the government's policies. Today, such groups make frequent demands for new NHI benefits, or for fee increases for certain services and procedures, or oppose premium rate increases, despite the decreasing share of government spending on the NHI and limited NHI premium revenue.

Members of organized interest groups have become a presence at the seat of governmental decision-making. Reportedly, it is a familiar sight in Taiwan's Parliament to see lobbyists accompany members of Parliament to hearings as observers, and chime in to question and criticize the government officials present. Some lobbyists even openly dispense instructions to legislators during session breaks (Tien, 2007).

The considerable involvement of organized interest groups and lobbyists in governmental decision-making is not in the best interests of patients, or supportive of efficient health care resource utilization. For example, after a lengthy period of consultation between the BNHI and physician groups, the BNHI has agreed to cover palliative care for terminal cancer patients in hospitals effective from January 2007 (Fang, 2006). Payment is on a per diem basis, thus setting a daily ceiling on the cost of treatments. Critics of the government's coverage decision point out that end-of-life care in hospital settings medicalizes the end-of-life process, where hospice care is commonly regarded (in other countries) as the preferred and more humane way to care for terminally ill patients. From the view point of best use of health care resources, coverage for palliative care in hospitals no doubt displaces other, perhaps more clinically efficacious, medical services for patients whose illnesses or conditions are amenable to medical interventions.

Another example of lobbying by interest groups in Taiwan came to light by way of a superior court case involving alleged political contributions made by the Taiwan Dentist Association (TDA) to numerous members of Parliament, both past and present, in its attempt to persuade Parliament to pass the oral hygiene bill into law. The TDA's objective was to save the oral hygiene services, which are a profitable part of dentists' practices and closely guarded dental "professional turf," from possible exclusion of insurance coverage by the proposed Second Generation NHI reform (G2 NHI Reform), currently pending in Parliament (Tien and Chen, 2007).

Recent Reforms, Options Considered, and Outcomes of Recent Reforms

As has been discussed earlier, the NHI has had financial difficulties ever since 1998, three years after its implementation in 1995. Since 1998, the NHI expenditure has consistently outpaced revenue by one to two percentage points. Most of the reform debates, therefore, have focused on the reform of the NHI's finances. Other debates centered on payments to providers, quality of care, equity issues, etc.

In the NHI's 14-year history, there has been but one premium rate increase, which took place in September 2002. At that time, the premium rate increase was calculated to restore and maintain the NHI's financial balance through December 2004. The government had hoped that it could again increase the premium rate in December 2004, as the NHI Law permits premium rate increases every two years, if needed. The government's expectation, however, was met with a stubborn no by the public following a three-day Civic Convention held in January 2005. The Civic Convention was a specially held public forum where representatives of the public met with scholars of health policy and government officials to discuss the NHI's future course. It concluded with the passing of a resolution, the now famous "Three No's": no premium rate increase, no copayment increase, and no cuts in benefits. The public and their political representatives believed that the BNHI should reduce waste and abuse before asking for an increase in the premium rate. Its hope for a premium rate increase dashed, the BNHI then embarked on a policy, in 2005, of "microadjustments" ("minor tinkering," or *wei tiao*) to generate new funds for the NHI. For example, the government raised tobacco taxes from NT$5 (US$0.15 per pack) to NT$10 (US$0.31 per pack) and held lottery sales. In addition, the government raised the ceilings for levying premiums on the salary and wages of certain population groups. For example, previously, 82.42% of the salary of public sector employees, including military personnel, was subject to premium contribution assessment; since 2005, 87.04% of their salary has been subject to premium contribution assessment (BNHI, 2006).

For some time now, the BNHI has found itself between a rock and a hard place. It faces, on the one hand, rising utilization driven by continuous introductions of superior technologies (like new drugs), rapid population aging, broadening of benefits for the care of people with serious diseases, and quality improvement measures. And, on the other hand, it faces the public and politicians' stubborn refusal to pay higher premium contributions, on the grounds that the NHI is beset by too much waste which should first be eliminated (Cheng, 2008). The experience of Taiwan confirms the findings of Pierson (1999) about the popularity of certain entitlements: once in place, entitlements of health care rapidly become popular and create their own constituencies. Thus, it is difficult for governments to delist entitlement or increase cost sharing for health care.

At this writing, the BNHI is borrowing from banks to pay for the shortfall in revenues. According to the former CEO of the BNHI, Chu Tzer-ming, every new day the NHI faces a new deficit of NT$70 million (US$2.15 million), which accumulates to NT$2 billion (US$61.44 million) per month. If things do not change, Chu expected the total 2008 deficit to be around NT$20 billion (US$614.4 million), or about 5% of the total annual expenditure of the NHI, the highest single-year deficit since the NHI's implementation (Shih and Tseng, 2008).

Financial troubles aside, the NHI faces numerous other challenges. By international standards, Taiwan's physian-population and nurse-population ratios are low. Figure 4 illustrates the ratio of physicians and nurses to the

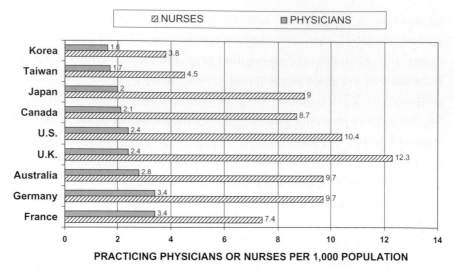

Source: (a) Department of Health. 2006. *2005 Health Statistical Trends*. Taipei: Department of Health, Executive Yuan. (2) OECD. 2008. *OECD Health Data*. Paris: OECD.

Fig. 4. Health workers per 1000 population in Taiwan and selected OECD countries, 2005.

greater population in Taiwan and select OECD countries in 2005 (DoH, 2006; OECD, 2008).

In addition, the length of a visit (time spent with the doctor during a visit) is short in Taiwan; anecdotes abound about the "three-minute visit." However, this phenomenon is not limited to Taiwan, and can be seen in China, Japan, and South Korea as well. Hospital emergency rooms are crowded; sometimes patients cannot get a bed at the more popular, higher-level hospitals, even after waiting three days in the hospital ER hall (Lin, 2008). Significant also, although hardly unique to Taiwan, is the problem of large variations in the quality of care among Taiwan's providers.

Workforce shortages in certain specialties, like OBGYN and general surgery, have developed in recent years because the BNHI fees for these specialties are relatively low and the risk of malpractice suits is high. By contrast, high-paying specialties such as cosmetic surgery, dermatology, and ear-nose-throat (ENT) are extremely popular among medical students and licensed physicians looking for a career change. Worst of all, from the viewpoint of quality and patient safety, is how some specialty associations have come to view the enhancement of their members' income-generating ability as their mandate. For example, The Association for Plastic Surgery in Taiwan, which currently has a membership of over 600 doctors, welcomes any licensed physician to join, regardless of his or her specialty training. To date, the association has held two courses in laser treatments and over 100 doctors have received certificates of completion. Among the association's members, in order of numbers from largest to smallest, are OBGYNs, general surgeons, dentists, family medicine doctors, orthopedic doctors, and pediatricians (Lee, 2006). Media reports of cosmetic surgery "mishaps" abound.

Also troublesome for Taiwan's champions of comprehensive, universal, and equitable health insurance is the increasing out-of-pocket spending by households, as patients are saddled with higher copayments, coinsurance, and registration fees to compensate for the NHI's financial deficit. According to Taiwan's Federation of NHI Public Oversight, a public interest NGO that serves as a watchdog on the overall operations of the NHI, hospitals and clinics in Taiwan have raised their registration fees by as much as 50% in the most recent two years, for a total aggregate collection of NT$50 billion (US$1.54 billion). That is close to one-eighth of the total annual NHI expenditure, which providers may keep because registration fees fall outside the NHI's domain. These high user fees have begun to create barriers to access for some patients (Lin, 2008). As of January 2008, registration fees charged by some primary care clinics can be as high as NT$400 (US$12). Not long ago, these fees averaged NT$50 (US$1.50) (Lin, 2008).

Finally, it appears that Taiwan may be developing a de facto private sector for wealthy patients. Physicians who are dissatisfied with the NHI's global budgets or want to earn higher pay than what the NHI provides as income have resorted to seeking profits from the sale of products and services that fall outside of the NHI's coverage or purview. For example, Taiwan's leading academic medical center, the National Taiwan University (*Taida*) Hospital, operates a private VIP clinic staffed by senior physicians with professorial ranks who see patients willing and able to pay the clinic's NT$1000 (US$31) registration fee. All other services, including diagnostic tests and drugs, are reimbursed by the BNHI according to its regular fee schedules. The Federation of NHI Public Oversight alleges that, in essence, a two-tiered system has been created, with access to the "best and brightest senior doctors" available to only those who can afford the NT$1000 registration fee. In other words, patients who cannot afford the higher fees do not have access to these same physicians. Taiwan's public perceives care provided by these senior doctors to be superior to that provided by more junior doctors, who may be junior in rank or are interns and residents (Wei, 2007). One is reminded in this instance of the "boutique" medicine that has sprung up in the U.S., where patients purchase superior round-the-clock access to physicians with an out-of-pocket annual retainer of anywhere from US$2000 to US$10,000.

In April 2008, talk of the long overdue premium rate increase was once again heard in Taiwan (Shih, 2008). The BNHI believes that the NHI's chronic financial troubles may be solved either by a premium rate increase or by enlarging the income base on which premiums are assessed and collected. Up until now, calculations for premium contributions are based only on wages and salaries — as in many other social insurance systems around the world. Other sources of income, such as rent, interest, and dividends, remain outside of the premium calculations. Many policy analysts in Taiwan believe that calculating premiums using the salary and wage alone as the base is neither equitable nor sufficient. Such a base favors wealthy individuals whose non-salary or wage incomes often far exceed their salary or wage. In addition, such a basis is simply too small to bear the ever-rising cost of health care. Wealthy individuals making incomes, in addition to, or in lieu of, their salary or wage should, in theory, pay higher premiums in a system whose financing is based on the principle of ability to pay. In Taiwan, however, such individuals have paid less in premiums than their wealth could have borne.

As noted earlier, the NHI premium rate has not been increased since the one and only increase in 2002. The rate increase of 7% in 2002 was a modest one. The rate increase proposed in the spring of 2008 by the BNHI would have increased the rate from the current 4.55% to 5.18%, an increase of 13.8% (Wei, 2008). Such an increase, if approved by Parliament, would have the greatest financial impact on the more than 12 million members of Taiwan's "salaried class." The assessable average monthly salary of this class is NT$32,000 (US$965), so the premium paid by a family of four would increase by NT$240 (US$7) per month, from NT$1748 (US$53) to NT$1988 (US$60) (Shih and Tseng, 2008).

According to estimates made by the former BNHI CEO and president, Chu Tzer-ming, a scholar in public finance, increasing the premium rate to 5.18% would produce an additional annual revenue of NT$40 billion (US$1.2 billion). It is hoped that this sum will be sufficient to keep a balanced budget plus one month's reserve for the NHI for the next five years (Shih and Tseng, 2008).

However, the best hope for the long-term financial future of Taiwan's NHI may lie in the campaign promise made by Taiwan's new president, Ma Ying-jeou, in November 2007, as the then presidential candidate of the KMT. Candidate Ma had promised to increase health care spending by up to 1.5% of GDP, from the current 6.2% to 7.5% or so of GDP. By OECD standards, taking into account Taiwan's per capita GDP, Taiwan's health spending is considerably below what it, in theory, could afford. Figure 5 shows the total national health spending as a percentage of GDP in Taiwan in 2007 and select OECD countries in 2006.

In the March 2008 presidential election, then candidate Ma Ying-jeou had the crucial and necessary support of Taiwan's medical community, mainly because the latter had been disappointed with how things had turned out for them under the previous government, led by the Democratic Progressive Party (DPP) (Lin, 2008). Perhaps the long-awaited "window of opportunity" is upon Taiwan's NHI once again and major reform may be possible in the next four to eight years.

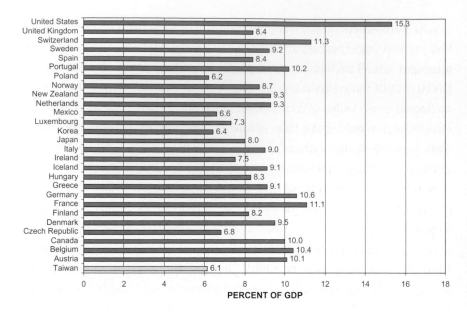

Fig. 5. NHE/GDP in OECD countries (2006) and Taiwan (2007).

Conclusion

For all of its many remarkable attributes and accomplishments, Taiwan's NHI exhibits the same Achilles heel that makes all government-run single-payer health systems vulnerable; namely, it must balance four sets of incompatible demands — those of health care providers, patients, citizens, and politicians.

Taiwan's health care providers view the NHI as a limitless source of financing for their income and professional aspirations, which, among providers of health care the world over, know few bounds. For their part, patients view the NHI as an institution that can and should finance whatever entitlement they and their doctors fancy, however reasonable or unreasonable these expectations may be. Citizens, as taxpayers and payers of premiums, resent the premium increases proposed by the BNHI because they believe that it countenances too much "fraud, waste, and abuse."

Finally, politicians everywhere pretend that eliminating "fraud, waste, and abuse" in health care would yield enough savings to finance the growing cost of truly needed health care, including new medical technology. In the U.S., that attitude has always stood as a barrier against extending health insurance to the uninsured; "cost control first, universal coverage later" has been the mantra. In Taiwan, the pretense is that the NHI would not be in financial difficulty if it managed to eliminate the "fraud, waste and abuse" in the system. In fact, of course, the "fraud, waste, and abuse" assumed to be in the system are incomes to the providers of health care. These providers are the same ones who hold considerable sway over the very politicians who, on the one hand, allege "fraud, waste, and abuse" but, on the other, more often than not, end up shielding such (waste) from serious cost reductions. Furthermore, it is not clear how much fraud, waste and abuse there actually are in health systems. To illustrate, if $100,000 or more is spent on a biological specialty drug to extend the life of a terminally ill patient by a month or two, is that "waste" or "needed care"?

Tax-financed government-run single-payer health systems require a certain degree of what one may call social patriotism, i.e. a willingness to forego the perfectly selfish conduct extolled in modern economic theory. The assumption is that providers of health care act responsibly and are willing to hold themselves openly accountable for their use of public funds. Patients must be reasonable in their demands on the health system. Politicians must lead the people with a vision of social solidarity, rather than cotton to the popularity of tax cuts or, in Taiwan's case, accept the "Three No's" as legitimate.

In the absence of such civic conduct, tax-financed single-payer systems will eventually show strains at the fringes, as is happening now in Canada. For one thing, there are long wait times in Canada for certain high-tech procedures, such as imaging, or certain elective surgical procedures. Furthermore, there is currently a debate in Canada on whether to allow a second, privately financed tier of health care to develop, parallel to the publicly financed one. Neither development has yet appeared on the scene in Taiwan, but they might. Proposals to privatize the financing of health care or to increase cost sharing by patients — called, euphemistically, putting their "skin in the game" — typically appeal to the ever-more-popular theory that most illnesses in modern society are lifestyle-induced. Using this argument, society's healthier and wealthier people may yearn to arrange for themselves, and finance with their own money, a better deal in health care than they wish to finance for everyone else with their tax dollars.

So far these social fissures have not yet manifested themselves in Taiwan's debate on health policy. Social solidarity in health care remains intact. But if Taiwan's policy-makers insist on keeping in place the current fiscal stranglehold on Taiwan's health system, that *nouvelle vague* may wash ashore in Taiwan as well. The next decade will tell.

References

Bureau of National Health Insurance. (2006). *National Health Insurance in Taiwan — Profile 2006*. Bureau of National Health Insurance, Taipei.

Bureau of National Health Insurance. (2006). *2005 National Health Insurance Profile*. Bureau of National Health Insurance, Taipei.

Bureau of National Health Insurance. (2007). *National Health Insurance in Taiwan — Profile 2007*. Bureau of National Health Insurance, Taipei.

Bureau of National Health Insurance. (2008). *A Profile of the National Health Insurance in Taiwan*. Chu Tzer-ming, Taipei.

Bureau of National Health Insurance. (2008). *Special Report to the 156th NHI Oversight Committee of the Department of Health: National Health Insurance Expenditures*. Bureau of National Health Insurance, Taipei.

Chang HJ. (2005). "Taiwan's National Health Insurance: Current Development and Performance." *Proceedings of Taiwan NHI's 10th Anniversary International Symposium*. Bureau of National Health Insurance, Taipei.

Cheng TM. (2003). "Taiwan's new National Health Insurance Program: Genesis and experience So Far." *Health Affairs* **22**(3): 61–76.

Cheng TM. (2007). Meetings with physicians and hospital administrators of National Taiwan University Hospital, Jen-Ai Municipal Hospital, Chang-Gung Memorial Hospital. Taipei.

Cheng TM. (2008). Meeting with Vice President CH Lee. Bureau of National Health Insurance, Taipei.

Cheng TM. (2008). "Taiwan's National Health Insurance: Lessons for the United States." Congressional briefing. US Congress, Washington, DC.

Cheng TM. (2008). "Taiwan's National Health Insurance: Lessons Learned and Future Challenges." Seminar, Princeton University.

Department of Health. (2005). *2004 Health Statistical Trends*. Department of Health, Executive Yuan, Taipei.

Department of Health. (2006). *2005 Health Statistical Trends*. Department of Health, Executive Yuan, Taipei.

Department of Health. (2007). *2006 Health Statistical Trends*. Department of Health, Executive Yuan, Taipei.

Department of Health. (2007). *2006 National Health Insurance Statistical Report*. Department of Health, Executive Yuan, Taipei.

Department of Health. (2008). *2007 Health Statistical Trends*. Department of Health, Executive Yuan, Taipei.

Department of Health. (2009). *2007 Health Statistical Trends*. Department of Health, Executive Yuan, Taipei.

Devlin N, Appleby J, Parkin D. (2003). "Patients' views of explicit rationing: What are the implications for health service decision-making?" *J Health Serv Res Policy* **8**: 183–186.

Fang KD. (2006). "Palliative care also made it into the ranks of covered NHI benefits." *Jian Kang Tai Wan Lun Tan* [Healthy Taiwan Forum]. Accessed 5 January 2009. http://blog.yam.com/healthy_taiwan.

International Monetary Fund. (2009). "EconoStats: IMF World Economic Outlook." Accessed 5 January 2009. http://econstats.com/weo/ CTWN.htm.

Lee SJ. (2006). "Dashing towards money goal: Pediatricians trained in cosmetic surgery." United Daily Evening News, 9 July.

LeGrand J. (2003). "Methods of cost containment: Some lessons from Europe." Lecture, Third International Health Economics Association World Congress, San Francisco.

Lin JY. (2008). "Registration fees earn NT$5 Yi a year; no way to control it." *United Daily Evening News*, 24 January.

Lin SM. (2008). "Health care moving towards M-curve: Regional hospitals survival in doubt." *United Daily News*, 25 April.

OECD. (2008). *OECD Health Data*. OECD, Paris.

Pedersen K. (2007). "Information technology in Taiwan's national health insurance." Panel remark, 5th International Health Economics Association World Congress, Copenhagen, Denmark, 10 July.

Peterson CL, Burton R. (2007). *CRS Report for Congress: U.S. Health Care Spending — Comparison with Other OECD Countries*. Domestic Social Policy Division, Congressional Research Service, Washington, DC.

Shih JR. (2008). "NHI premium rate hike heard: NHI's heavy financial burden raises fear of rise in 'NHI comorbidity.'" *United Daily News*, 26 April.

Shih JR, Tseng JR. (2008). "Proposed NHI premium rate increase: Monthly payment for family of four to increase by NT$240." *United Daily News*, 26 April.

Tien SM, Chen ST. (2007). "Interest groups shuttling back and forth in Parliament brazenly." *Liberty Times*, 18 July.

Wei LW. (2007). "Tiring of patient access: Rich receive VIP- and poor poor treatments." *United Daily News*, 27 July.

Wei LW. (2008). "Bureau of National Health Insurance looks to premium rate hike: No time set for implementation." *United Daily News*, 26 April.

Yeh CC. (2002). *The Legend of the National Health Insurance*. The Tung Foundation, Taipei.

Yeh CC. (2007). *The NHI Walking with You Hand in Hand*. Bureau of National Health Insurance, Taipei.

Conclusions: Debates, Reforms, and Policy Adjustments

Kieke G. H. Okma and Luca Crivelli

This chapter summarizes our findings on the origins and fates of the health reform efforts in six small and midsize democracies — Israel, The Netherlands, New Zealand, Singapore, Switzerland, and Taiwan — in the 1980s and 1990s.

Why did these countries embark on the health reform trail? What were the major policy goals and reform options discussed? Was there explicit reference to other countries' experiences? Who were the main stakeholders and what were their positions? What option became reality? What actually happened during implementation? And, finally, what were the (intended and unintended, expected and unexpected) outcomes?

In the 1980s and 1990s, all six countries undertook systematic reviews of their health care systems, spurred by budgetary and fiscal restraints, evolving ideologies, and changing economic realities. Indeed, the combined effects of the oil crises in the mid-1970s, the end of the postwar baby boom, and changing ideological views regarding the role of the state versus citizens triggered extensive debate about the future of welfare states as a whole. The exceptions were Singapore and Taiwan, where long periods of high economic growth and budget surpluses in the 1980s and 1990s enabled the rapid and smooth passage of new policies. Singapore's and Taiwan's newfound prosperity not only raised their populations' expectations of the government's role in initiating income protection schemes against the financial risks of old age and illness, but also provided the fiscal means for ensuring that the entire population could benefit. Capitalizing on these periods of phenomenal economic growth, those two "Asian tigers" realized universal health coverage via expansion, rather than contraction, of the welfare state, though in strikingly different ways.

In all the six countries studied, the goals of the reforms — at least rhetorically — were similar: improved access to health services (through expanding public or private health insurance), improved quality and efficiency of services (through a mix of market-oriented and regulatory measures), overall cost control, and greater consumer and patient choice (freedom to switch to another insurer, or to a different health plan, but also free choice of provider). All countries realized universal or near-universal health coverage, but their success with other goals, in particular cost control and consumer choice, has been more modest. The insured now have a greater choice of health insurer (or health plan) in Switzerland, the Netherlands, and Israel, but, simultaneously, the introduction of selective contracting by health insurers has actually reduced patients' choice of provider in Switzerland and The Netherlands. In those countries, insurers have gained decision-making power over contracting with providers. In several countries, governments imposed restrictions on health care insurers and providers, while the Taiwan government became the sole health insurer itself. The expansion of private insurance led to increased risk selection in Switzerland and The Netherlands. Indeed, shifts toward decentralized private governance also increased the administrative complexity and overhead costs in those countries.

The more centralized systems have been more successful in realizing the goal of cost containment because of uniform administration and the imposition of countrywide fees and tariffs. The administrative and political complexity of the Swiss model is reflected in its rising costs; a few years after the introduction of the 1996 reforms, Switzerland was surpassed only by the U.S. in health spending. The 2006 Health Insurance Law in The Netherlands did not lead to improved cost control, either.

At the ends of the health care governance spectrum are full nationalization and full privatization of health insurance and provision. Ultimately, no country fully privatized or fully nationalized its entire health care system. Israel extended its Bismarckian model of employment-based insurance to cover the entire population, but left the responsibility for administering the scheme in the hands of the existing sick funds. It also introduced choice of fund for the insured. Singapore, despite 140 years of British rule and influence, never went "Beveridgean" (universal tax-based health care), but instead emphasized individual over state responsibility and encouraged private sector participation. At the same time, low-income families receive state subsidy for their savings accounts and hospital stays, and the government has maintained a stringent role in overall program design, as well as other controls. After carefully considering alternatives, Taiwan incorporated and extended existing schemes into one population-wide health insurance. New Zealand moved toward a more commercial and competitive model for its public health system during the 1990s, but reverted to a more traditional public sector model after the election of a Labour-led government in 1999. Over four decades, The Netherlands reform debate shifted from considering a fully nationalized health insurance with state-controlled health care provision (based on regional planning) toward market-oriented options. In 2006, it implemented a new insurance model that, like Switzerland's, combines public and private elements. Switzerland took the lead in experimenting with a new health insurance model that combined public rules with private insurance administration. The 1996 law requires that all residents take out health insurance with legally defined basic coverage, with the possibility of choosing alternative plans with different financial conditions. It maintained the mix of public and private (for-profit and not-for-profit) providers.

Not only the direction but also the speed of implementing reforms varied widely. For example, in the mid-1990s, after carefully considering alternatives, Taiwan opted for a nationwide public health insurance scheme, by far the simplest model for universal coverage and uniform administration (and, as experience elsewhere has shown, the model with the lowest administrative costs). It implemented the model in a remarkably short time span. With similar speed, Singapore put in place a complicated mix of private (but mandatory) savings schemes and public safety net funding. It successfully implemented an ingenious financing mechanism that, combined with public subsidies for primary and hospital care, ensures that everyone has access to basic medical services. Singapore first wanted to privatize all of its hospitals, but, faced with public dissatisfaction, the government rapidly reversed its course and kept public hospitals and other health facilities under government ownership and control. With hospital restructuring, the quality of care improved, but it came at higher costs. New Zealand, too, completely restructured its public health system within two years by separating the purchase and provision of health services. However, its basic (tax-based) funding model remained unchanged.

Singapore exemplifies "exclusionary policy-making", where strong central governments can design and implement (and rapidly adjust) major policy change without much opposition from organized interests. Similarly, Taiwan's one-party dominance allowed for rapid change, though in recent years Taiwan has experienced a rise in political opposition and citizen empowerment that has slowed policy change in some cases. Governments of countries with "older" models of "inclusionary" policy-making in place, like Israel or The Netherlands, have had a much harder time fundamentally changing their system in the face of opposing stakeholders. In fact, both Israel and The Netherlands (and, to a lesser degree, Switzerland) have neocorporatist policy legacies, where governments share the responsibility for social policy-making with organized stakeholders. That tradition provides ample veto power to stakeholders anxious to prevent change that would negatively affect their positions. Israel and The Netherlands also have long traditions of multiparty coalition governments that create the need for compromise; such compromise can slow processes of policy-making, but it also contributes to political stability.

Organized citizens or patients did not play a dominant role in shaping the reform process in any of the countries in this study, though governments often quoted expanding consumer and patient choice as one of the main reasons for implementing change. In several cases, broad popular support for existing social policy severely restrained the governments' attempts to shift costs to patients, or forced policy-makers to adjust their course.

All countries have shifted, or are in the process of shifting, payment for hospital care from overall global budgets or per diem payments to some form of diagnoses-related groups (DRGs) or case-based payment. It is important to note that the shape and actual application of DRGs vary across countries. For example, New Zealand uses DRGs as a basis for estimating the global budgets based on volumes and prices. Strictly speaking, those are not case-based payments, but rather payments based on DRGs. The DRG model rarely covers all expenses, as hospitals often receive separate funding for their capital investments and certain very expensive treatments. In several countries, the introduction of the DRG model turned out to be more complicated and time-consuming than policy-makers had expected (or hoped). In all countries, self-employed health professionals receive fees for their services, often combined with additional payment for specific activities. There is great variation in payment of medical specialists, ranging from salaried physicians in New Zealand hospitals to hospital-based or fully independent practitioners with long-term contracts with hospitals and health insurers in other countries. Instead of fully shifting from one payment model to another, all countries moved toward mixed payment methods for medical care.

Some countries studied the experiences abroad before deciding on their reform course. Both Singapore and Taiwan explicitly "shopped around" for health reform ideas and considered a variety of experiences abroad as possible options before finally implementing two entirely different models. Conversely, in The Netherlands, the 1987 "Dekker Committee" report has no references to other countries' experiences. However, in the early 2000s, Dutch policy-makers and politicians visited Switzerland and were clearly impressed with what they saw (or wanted to see), and The Netherlands' 2006 Health Insurance Law resembles the Swiss model (but without the restraints of devolved administration).

One common phenomenon is that the labels used in international debate do not always reflect reality. For example, Singapore is often characterized as the country that successfully introduced individual savings accounts to pay for medical care, but in fact those accounts contribute only a very modest share of total health care funding. Direct patient payments, government subsidy, and employers' mandatory contributions account for a much bigger share of total funding. Moreover, the Singapore government provides several forms of cross-subsidies to safeguard access to health care for lower-income groups. Additionally, Dutch governments initially labeled the proposals for the 2006 health insurance scheme as "private," but for different reasons it eventually became known as "public."

What are the lessons we can draw from these experiences?

First, major change is rare. However, the cases of this study confirm that political and other events can combine to create "windows of opportunity" (Kingdon, 1984) that allow entrepreneurial politicians and policymakers to propose and implement major change. For example, the confluence of political willingness (and power) to change, popular perceptions of the need to reform, and the availability of reform options that fit the national context created a fertile ground for Taiwan and Singapore to successfully implement major reforms. In The Netherlands, the erosion of some of the institutions that traditionally dominated social policy-making (and that offered ample opportunity for organized stakeholders to block change), combined with the return of the Christian Democratic Party as the dominant coalition party in the early 2000s, allowed for the surprisingly rapid passage of a reform law in 2006. Israel shares some of the neocorporatist features of the social policy arena with Germany, Switzerland, and The Netherlands. This model has traditionally provided organized interests with veto power to thwart or slow change proposed by the government, or to limit the range of policy options. For example, the 2006 reform in The Netherlands reflected as much long-term continuity as change in health policy, the federalist politics in Switzerland blocked efforts to implement a more centralized governance of social health insurance, and, in Israel, organized stakeholders prevented the government from fully implementing the planned reforms.

Second, values matter. Dominant cultural orientations or values in society contribute to the shaping of political and other institutions that serve to channel interests; conversely, these institutions shape values. As we have observed elsewhere, values can channel policy-making in a certain direction, or exclude certain options, but they do not tell policy-makers exactly what to do (Marmor, Okma, and Latham, 2006). In general, values do not change quickly. For example, in many countries there is strong popular support for old age pension schemes and government-sponsored (but not necessarily government-provided) health care (perhaps even more than for unemployment and disability benefits). When the New Zealand government tried to introduce a competitive model in the 1990s, health professionals felt totally alienated and forced the government to move back to a more cooperative model in the 2000s. Almost every-where, strong popular support for government-sponsored arrangements that safeguard universal access to health care has limited governments' options to shift too much of the financial burden to families. In this respect, Singapore is a rare exception: an entitlement culture has not taken root. The government has coaxed the highly disciplined, rags-to-riches immigrant population into assuming greater responsibility for its own health care. Mitigated by government subsidies, health care financing has shifted to private pockets without much fuss. Singapore's Medisave scheme appealed to traditional Asian values by identifying the family, rather than the state, as the basic unit of solidarity and risk pooling.

Third, institutions matter. In a narrow sense, political institutions, defined as the political decision-making structure, are crucial for enabling not only reform but also speed in change, like in Singapore and Taiwan. In contrast, the particular institutional configuration of the Swiss federalist tradition has limited the range of options available to policy-makers. In a wider sense, "institutions" include not only political traditions but also other organizations (and generally accepted practices) in societies that contribute to the shaping and outcome of social policy. In this broader sense, institutions have been important in explaining slow policy change in Israel and The Netherlands, where powerful stakeholders thwart or slow reform efforts. Certain policies, once in place, can create their own constituencies (Pierson, 1994). For example, old age pension schemes and social health insurance have become popular in many countries. The experience in The Netherlands and elsewhere shows that beneficiaries (in the case of health care, patients, their families, and providers) will resist increasing patient cost-sharing, delisting entitlements, or other attempts to shift the financial burden from the government to citizens.

Fourth, reforming health care systems is not a one-shot effort. Most countries have adjusted their reform pathways when outcomes did not meet expectations. In all cases, there was a need for "postreform maintenance." Facing public dissatisfaction and strong opposition from organized stakeholders, governments had to adjust their policy course or abandon policies altogether. In fact, postreform maintenance seems to be a more or less permanent feature everywhere. Both endogenous and exogenous factors contribute to this process of permanent change. Government policy is a major force in the health policy arena, but it is not the only one. For example, innovation in medical technology has improved the quality of care and expanded treatment options (while also driving up costs). New managerial ideas and information technology affect the organization and governance of hospitals and health facilities. The main actors in the health system often adjust or try to gain strategic positions as they anticipate new realities. External fiscal strains and budgetary pressures restrict the availability of public funding. Moreover, unexpected and undesired policy outcomes may force governments to adjust their course or reverse earlier steps.

Fifth, attempts to categorize countries are inevitably flawed. It is hard, if not impossible, to design or apply any meaningful categorization of countries or their entire health care systems. Countries face similar challenges and options, but differ greatly in the direction and speed of implementing social policy change because of country-specific contextual factors. This study presents common problems and policy options, common system elements, and a common range of policy instruments and measures considered, but there is no clear overall pattern in the constellation of those system elements before or after the health reforms. It thus may be more important to focus on system elements than on entire countries or "health care systems"; it is easier to categorize (or characterize) programs and policies than an entire country's health arrangements. This level of analysis offers a more realistic laboratory of policy change than (announced) health system reform at the national level. For example, the slow implementation of DRG-based payment in Israeli and Dutch hospitals contrasts with the rapid speed of introducing similar change in Singapore (where DRG payments took only one year to roll out). Israel's successful experience with defining the entitlements of the social health insurance (or "explicit rationing") stands out as a specific policy experience not shared by other countries (even while other countries have faced this same issue).

Finally, despite the rhetoric of retrenchment, consumer choice, and market competition, there has been more, rather than less, government action almost everywhere. Nowhere did governments give up their regulatory authority over health care, even in cases where they strongly supported markets and consumer choice as instruments for allocating resources. Some countries developed new instruments for monitoring markets and informing consumers, but kept old ones in place for controlling public (and sometimes private) expenditure, for example by delisting entitlements from social insurance, and by imposing budgets, user fees, and changes in payment methods.

Appendix A: Statistical Data — Israel, The Netherlands, New Zealand, Singapore, Switzerland, and Taiwan

Table 1 presents statistical data on the size and populations of the six countries of this study. It shows that in terms of size, New Zealand is the largest country of the group and Singapore the smallest, even while their populations are almost equal. The population density is by far the highest in Singapore, followed by that of The Netherlands and then of Israel. In all the countries concerned, over two-thirds of the population live in urban areas.

Table 2 provides data on income and economic growth rates in the 1980s, 1990s, and early 2000s. Switzerland has the highest average income, with The Netherlands and Singapore second and third. The lowest is Taiwan. However, measured in Purchasing Power Parity (PPP), the differences in income are much smaller than when measured in current dollar amounts. This also applies to health spending (see Table 3). It is important to take real family incomes into account when comparing levels of health spending between countries.

Table 3 compares the levels of health spending in the six countries of this study. Switzerland has the highest levels of health expenditure (expressed as share of gross domestic product, GDP), as well as the highest spending per capita, followed by that of The Netherlands. Singapore has both the lowest spending levels and amounts of current dollars, followed by that of Taiwan. Again, as seen in Table 2, it is important to take the relative purchasing powers of national currencies into account: when expressed in Purchasing Power Parity, the difference in health spending between countries is much smaller than in current U.S. dollar amounts.

Table 1. Country Size and Populations of Israel, The Netherlands, New Zealand, Singapore, Switzerland, and Taiwan

	Size (1000 sq. km)	Population, 2008 (millions)	Population Density, 2008 (people/sq. km)	Population in Urban Areas, 2006 (%)
Israel	22	7.1	342.4	92
The Netherlands	42	16.6	400.8	81
New Zealand	268	4.2	15.5	86
Singapore	0.7	4.6	6652.5	100
Switzerland	41	7.6	183.6	76
Taiwan	36	22.9	637.1	63.2*

*2005

Sources: Central Intelligence Agency, 2008, "CIA World Factbook" <https://www.cia.gov/library/publications/the-world-factbook/index.html>. Department of Health, Republic of China, 2006, "2005 Public Health Report," Taiwan: Department of Health, R.O.C. World Health Organization, 2009, "WHO Statistical Information System" <http://www.who.int/whosis/en/index.html>.

Table 2. Income Levels and Economic Growth in Israel, The Netherlands, New Zealand, Singapore, Switzerland, and Taiwan

	GDP Per Capita, 2007 (US$)	GDP Per Capita, 2008 (PPP)	GDP Growth, 1980–1990 (%)	GDP Growth, 1990–1999 (%)	GDP Growth, 2000–2004 (%)
Israel	23,383	28,900	3.6	5.3	1.0
The Netherlands	46,669	41,300	2.2	2.9	0.5
New Zealand	31,219	28,500	1.9	3.2	4.0
Singapore	36,370	52,900	7.4	7.7	2.9
Switzerland	56,579	40,900	2.2	1.0	0.6
Taiwan	15,036*	33,000	NA	8.7	3.5

*2004

Sources: Central Intelligence Agency, 2008, "CIA World Factbook" <https://www.cia.gov/library/publications/the-world-factbook/index.html>. Department of Health, Republic of China, 2006, "2005 Public Health Report," Taiwan: Department of Health, R.O.C. United Nations, 2009, "United Nations Statistics Division" <http://unstats.un.org/unsd/default.htm>. World Bank, 2006, *World Development Indicators 2006*, Washington: The World Bank.

Table 4 summarizes a few core health care inputs (including the number of physicians and hospital beds) and health status measures (life expectancy and child mortality). These data sets confirm what has been shown time and again by other studies: life expectancy or child

Table 3. Health Care Spending in Israel, The Netherlands, New Zealand, Singapore, Switzerland, and Taiwan

	Total Health Expenditure, 2000 (% of GDP)	Total Health Expenditure, 2005 (% of GDP)	Share of Public Health Spending, 2000 (%)	Share of Public Health Spending, 2004 (%)	Per Capita Total Health Expenditure, 2000 (US$)	Per Capita Total Health Expenditure, 2005 (US$)	Per Capita Total Health Expenditure, 2000 (PPP)	Per Capita Total Health Expenditure, 2005 (PPP)
Israel	8.0	7.8	71.8	70.0	1589	1533	1810	2143
The Netherlands	8.0	9.2	63.1	62.4	1925	3560	2337	3187
New Zealand	8.1	8.9	78.0	78.3	1109	2403	1686	2223
Singapore	3.4	3.5	35.4	34.0	790	944	874	1140
Switzerland	10.3	11.4	55.6	58.5	3572	5694	3256	4088
Taiwan	5.7	6.2*	60.6	64.2	794	908*	NA	NA

* 2004

Sources: OECD Health Data 2005; Taiwan Department of Health and Office of Statistics, 2006, "National Health Expenditures 2004," Taiwan: Department of Health, R.O.C. World Health Organization, 2009, "WHO Statistical Information System" <http://www.who.int/whosis/en/index.html>.

Note: It is important to note that the OECD and WHO data list the premiums for the mandatory health insurance in Switzerland and The Netherlands under "public spending." Conceptually, these premiums might be labeled private, as they are administered by private health insurers (see footnote 8, chapter on The Netherlands).

Table 4. Health Care Resources and Health Status of Populations in Israel, The Netherlands, New Zealand, Singapore, Switzerland, and Taiwan

	Physician Density, 2000–2003[+] (Per 1000 Population)	Health Worker Density Index, 2000–2003[+] (Per 1000 Population)	Hospital Bed Density, 2002–2008[+] (Per 1000 Population)	Life Expectancy at Birth, 1980 (Years)	Life Expectancy at Birth, 2008 (Years)	Infant Mortality, 1980 (Per 1000 Live Births)	Infant Mortality, 2008 (Per 1000 Live Births)
Israel	3.8	10.3	6.0	73.9	80.6	16.1	4.3
The Netherlands	3.1	16.7	5.0	76.7	79.2	8.7	4.8
New Zealand	2.2	10.9	6.0	73.4	80.2	13.0	4.9
Singapore	1.5	5.6	3.2	71.5	81.9	11.7	2.3
Switzerland	3.6	12.1	5.7	75.5	80.7	9.1	4.2
Taiwan	1.4	4.4	6.7	69.6	77.8	8.0**	5.5
OECD average	3.0*	NA	5.5	72.5	78.9	17.9	5.2

[+] Data are for the most recent year available.

* 2004

** 1990

Sources: Central Intelligence Agency, 2008, "CIA World Factbook" <https://www.cia.gov/library/publications/the-world-factbook/index.html>. Department of Health, Republic of China, 2006, "Health Care Statistical Trends;" Taiwan: Department of Health, R.O.C. Government Information Office, Republic of China, 2008, "The Republic of China Yearbook 2008" <http://www.gio.gov.tw/taiwan-website/5-gp/yearbook/home.html>. OECD Health Data 2005. OECD Health Data 2008. World Bank, 2006, *World Development Indicators 2006*, Washington: The World Bank. World Health Organization, 2009.

mortality — commonly taken as measures of the quality of health care — are not closely related to spending levels for health care or number of health professionals. All countries saw the average life expectancy of the population increase, with the biggest increase in Singapore. Similarly, changes in child mortality rates show striking variation, with the largest decrease in Israel.

Table 5 summarizes the "dominant cultural orientations" and underlying welfare principles of the six countries in this study. These underlying values or orientations in society also find expression in their general fiscal, macro-economic, and social policies. Interestingly, there seems to be more similarities in health policies (see footnotes about "welfare principles") across countries than in other fields of social policy, perhaps reflecting the wide popular support for universal and solidaristic access to health care (and pensions). But over time, there have been policy shifts toward greater emphasis on market competition and individual responsibility in several countries. These shifts reflect long-term changes in underlying societal values, or social "climate changes," that have allowed governments to pass measures that would have once been considered unacceptable.

Table 6 summarizes the core characteristics in funding, contracting, ownership, and administration of health care. In most countries, public funding (general taxation and public health insurance) is the main funding source. In general, countries with higher income levels have lower shares of patient co-payments. Most, if not all, countries have sought to more clearly separate the functions of provision and funding of health services (the "purchaser-provider split"), but not all have abandoned the mandatory contracting by third party payers. This split has strengthened the role of independent (both non-profit and for-profit) health providers and third payers and confirms earlier findings of a common trend towards the "public contracting model" — the model that combines public funding with independent status of health care providers (OECD 1992, 1994). Reflecting wider change in public policy, there has been a decline in collective bargaining in some countries, notably The Netherlands, but in others, like Taiwan, the role of organized interests seems to be on the rise. The particular governance models are associated with varying degrees of consumer (and patient) "voice," "choice," and "exit" (see Introduction).

Table 7 summarizes some of the main events and features of health care systems that have created windows of opportunity for change in the countries of this study. It also shows the different constellations — and an interesting variety — of voice, choice, and exit options for patients and consumers in those systems.

Table 5. Dominant Cultural Orientation and Welfare Principles in Israel, The Netherlands, New Zealand, Singapore, Switzerland, and Taiwan

	Dominant Cultural Orientations and Welfare Principles in Fiscal, Macro-economic, and Social Policy	Dominant Values in Health Policy
Israel	Long tradition of employment-based income protection and (collectivist) solidarity in social policy; since 1980s, strong opposition to efforts to shift towards residualism; weak sectarianism	Strong solidarity and income protection; expansion of employment-based health insurance to universal coverage; universal access to broad range of health services
The Netherlands	Strong (but declining since 1980s) hierarchical collectivism (neo-corporatism); long tradition of employment-based income protection based on mix of public and private arrangements; since 1980s, shift towards more residualist social policy; weak sectarianism	Long tradition of employment-based health insurance; since 2006, individual mandate for all to take out (private) health insurance, with cross subsidy for lower income groups; efforts to de-list entitlements or increase co-payments restrained by solidaristic culture
New Zealand	Strong (but somewhat declining) collectivism; after economic policy change in 1990s, shift to residualist role of state in social policy; fairly strong sectarianism	Strong support for solidarity and income protection in health care; universal health insurance; universal access to broad range of health services (but traditionally excluding primary care)
Singapore	Strong emphasis on markets, competition, and individual and family responsibility; residualist role of state in social policy; acceptance of strong central government; weak sectarianism	Combination of individualistic and residualist policy with universal access health insurance and broad range of health services; tax-based subsidy for lower income groups

(Continued)

Table 5. *(Continued)*

	Dominant Cultural Orientations and Welfare Principles in Fiscal, Macro-economic, and Social Policy	Dominant Values in Health Policy
Switzerland	Liberal country with a certain tradition of social policy within decentralized federalism; since the mid-1990s, some shift of political power from the regional to the central state in the healthcare sector; general claim of a more residual role of state and greater emphasis on markets and competition; weak sectarianism	Long tradition of social employment-based insurance combined with individualist private health insurance; shift towards universal mandate to take private insurance with free choice of plan and provider
Taiwan	Residualist role of state in social policy; emphasis on individual rights and duties; emphasis on markets and competition; acceptance of strong role of government; weak sectarianism	Combination of individualistic and residualist policy, with (state-run) universal health insurance and universal access to broad range of health services

Sources: Authors.

Table 6. Funding, Contracting, Ownership, and Administration of Health Care in Israel, The Netherlands, New Zealand, Singapore, Switzerland, and Taiwan

	Main Funding Sources for Health Care	Contracting and Payment	Ownership and Governance of Health Care
Israel	General taxation (46%), health tax (29%), private payment (29%) 100% of population covered by social health insurance; 20% has supplemental coverage	Four competing sick funds contract with hospitals; paid by mix of per diem and case-based payment, with budget caps; outpatient care mostly fee-for-services	Dominance of public hospitals and public health services (about 50%); largest sick fund, Clalit, owns 30% of the other hospitals and private clinics; some private for-profit clinics Long tradition of strong stakeholder involvement and inclusionary policy-making; recently some decline of neo-corporatist collective bargaining
The Netherlands	Income-related earmarked taxation plus community-rated flat-rate premiums for health insurance (plus fiscal subsidy for low-income families); modest amounts of patient co-payments; voluntary supplemental insurance	Insures selectively contract with providers; mix of per diem and case-based payment, with budget caps for hospitals; some integrated contracting (local public health services); non-hospital care mix of capitation, fee-for-services, and special payments; selective contracting	Independent, mostly not-for-profit hospitals; recent rise of for-profit clinics; local public health clinics; self-employed professionals in primary care

(Continued)

Table 6. (*Continued*)

	Main Funding Sources for Health Care	Contracting and Payment	Ownership and Governance of Health Care
	100% of population has to take out insurance		Decline of neo-corporatist bargaining, but still strong stakeholder involvement in inclusionary policy-making
New Zealand	Universal, tax-based health care; modest amount of patient co-payments	Hospitals receive mix of per diem and case-based payment, with budget caps; outpatient care mostly fee-for-services; no selective contracting for hospital care	Hospitals publicly owned and funded. No tradition of neo-corporatist collective bargaining or inclusionary policy-making; stakeholder involvement in policy-making mostly via the political arena
	100% of population is automatically covered		
Singapore	Universal coverage based on mix of mandatory medical savings accounts, insurance, and targeted tax-based subsidies, with high out of pocket payments	Hospitals receive mix of per diem and case-based payment, with budget caps; outpatient care mostly fee-for-services; no selective contracting for hospital care	Hospital under government control, with some administrative independence; plans to expand private hospital capacity; outpatient care mainly by independent health professionals

(*Continued*)

Table 6. (*Continued*)

	Main Funding Sources for Health Care	Contracting and Payment	Ownership and Governance of Health Care
	100% of population has access to health care		No tradition of collective bargaining or organized stakeholder involvement in policy-making
Switzerland	Complex financing mix: community-based premiums for mandatory health insurance, federal and cantonal allowances for households with modest incomes, and direct subsidies from the regional and local governments for inpatient care; high out of pocket spending	Hospitals receive mix of per diem and case-based payment, some with budget caps; outpatient care mostly fee-for-services; no selective contracting	Mix of independent, not-for-profit hospitals and private clinics, independent health professionals in outpatient care
	100% of population has to take out insurance		Decline of neo-corporatist collective bargaining; strong stakeholder involvement in policy-making

(*Continued*)

Table 6. *(Continued)*

	Main Funding Sources for Health Care	Contracting and Payment	Ownership and Governance of Health Care
Taiwan	Universal public health insurance out of general taxation, with low (but rising) out of pocket spending.	Hospitals receive mix of per diem and case-based payment, with budget caps; outpatient care mostly fee-for-services; no selective contracting for hospital care	Public hospitals; independent health professionals in outpatient care
	100% of population is automatically covered		Public administration of health insurance; no tradition of neo-corporatist collective bargaining, but recent efforts to strengthen stakeholder involvement in policy-making

Sources: Authors.

Table 7. Windows of Opportunity and Voice, Choice, and Exit in Health Care in Israel, The Netherlands, New Zealand, Singapore, Switzerland, and Taiwan

	Window of Opportunity for Change	Voice, Choice and Exit in Health Care
Israel	Lack of public and political support created barriers for fully implementing reform proposals (some elements did pass); perhaps there was a "partial window" opened by confluence of fiscal and budgetary problems and political willingness to act (but proposed solution turned out not acceptable)	Four major sick funds "capture" the entire population, but patients have ample choice of provider as the long tradition of social insurance (with free choice of provider) limited options of selective contracting or market-oriented solutions. Low exit in the health insurance market; voice via the political channels
The Netherlands	Decades of health reform debate and partial implementation of Dekker proposals had already changed the positions and attitudes of major stakeholders, thus supporting market-oriented change that was unacceptable two decades earlier; after 8 years of exile, Christian Democrats returned to power, eager to act and presenting rapidly increasing health expenditure as evidence of urgent need to change	In theory, the 2006 universal scheme (mandate to take out private insurance) offers increased "exit" to consumers. In general, there is not much interest to change health plans, or health providers, with the exception of the popular cash benefit scheme for long-term care. Patient and consumer groups continue to express their voice as active advocates in health care

(Continued)

Table 7. (*Continued*)

	Window of Opportunity for Change	Voice, Choice and Exit in Health Care
New Zealand	After the economic recession of the 1980s had prompted governments to enact economic major restructuring, it also tried its hand with notions of internal markets found in the British NHS. Changing governing coalitions in 1993 and in 2000 combined with lack of structural veto points facilitated structural health reforms. However, lack of public support forced the new coalition government (no longer solo decision-maker) to undo some of the reforms	Traditionally, direct patient and consumer influence (voice) in social policy-making in NZ is limited as the assumption is that their interests are represented in the political process and in community representation in governing boards. Efforts to increase patient choice (exit) did not gain much support
Singapore	Rising incomes and public expectations, weak political opposition and the unique situation of budget surpluses gave the strong political leadership the opportunity to rapidly and pragmatically implement (and adjust) change	Singapore has little tradition of direct voice, but as the government has been successful in delivering on its promise to provide access to health care for all, it has met with high approval ratings. Patients have virtually unlimited access to health services, but have to pay more for extra amenities and better quality of service
Switzerland	After 85 years with little change in health insurance regulation (several popular votes ended up with the status quo), the confluence of agreement amongst major political parties and broad perceptions of	Swiss citizens have a unique degree of both voice and exit in health care. They have free choice of health plan, free choice of provider, and can also express preferences via the popular vote

(*Continued*)

Table 7. (*Continued*)

	Window of Opportunity for Change	Voice, Choice and Exit in Health Care
	malfunctioning of the old system opened a window of opportunity in 1994 when the new insurance law was passed by popular ballot with slight majority. The particular combination of a solid tradition of social insurance with free choice of provider, and political preference for market solutions led to the hybrid model of an universal mandate to take out (private) health insurance, with fiscal subsidy for low-income families	
Taiwan	Similar to Singapore, rising incomes and public expectations combined with strong political leadership willing and able to act quickly to impose the "best model" of state-administered, single payer universal health insurance	Like Singapore, Taiwan has had little tradition of direct patient or citizen influence in health care, but in recent years that has changed as the government has sought to enlarge their voice. The universal health insurance has also broadened patient choice of provider

Sources: Authors.

Index